# KIDNEY DISEASE DIET FOR STAGE 4

The Ultimate low in sodium, phosphorus and potassium easy-to-make Recipes Cookbook and Meal Plan to Improve Renal health and enhance healthy living.

Olivia Endwell

## Copyright Statement:

All rights reserved. No part of this publication may be reproduced, distributed, or transmitted in any form or by any means, including photocopying, recording, or other electronic or mechanical methods, without the prior written permission of the publisher, except in the case of brief quotations embodied in critical reviews and certain other noncommercial uses permitted by copyright law.

Olivia Endwell, 2024.

## Disclaimer:

The information provided in this book is for educational and informational purposes only. It is not intended as a substitute for professional medical advice, diagnosis, or treatment. Always seek the advice of your physician or other qualified health provider with any questions you may have regarding a medical condition. Never disregard professional medical advice or delay in seeking it because of something you have read in this book.

The author and publisher disclaim any liability arising directly or indirectly from the use of this book. The information provided is based on the author's best knowledge at the time of writing and is subject to change. The author and publisher do not guarantee the accuracy, completeness, or timeliness of the information presented in this book.

Individual results may vary, and the success of any dietary or lifestyle change depends on various factors, including but not limited to individual commitment and adherence. Before making significant changes to your diet or lifestyle, consult with a qualified healthcare professional.

The views and opinions expressed in this book are those of the author and do not necessarily reflect the official policy or position of any other agency, organization, employer, or company.

# TABLE OF CONTENTS

INTRODUCTION .................................................................................... 1

The Basics of a Kidney friendly Diet .................................................... 3

    Nutritional Requirements for Stage 4 Kidney Disease ................ 3

    Protein Intake ................................................................................ 4

    Sodium Restriction ........................................................................ 5

    Phosphorus and Potassium Management .................................... 6

Sodium and Fluid Control ...................................................................... 8

    Understanding Sodium's Impact .................................................... 8

    Hidden Sodium in Foods ............................................................... 9

    Fluid Intake Guidelines ................................................................. 10

    Balancing Hydration ..................................................................... 11

    Monitoring Fluid Levels ................................................................ 12

Managing Phosphorus and Potassium ................................................. 14

    Impact of Phosphorus and Potassium on Kidney Health ............ 14

    Phosphorus-Rich Foods ............................................................... 15

    Potassium-Rich Foods ................................................................. 16

    Strategies for Phosphorus and Potassium Control .................... 17

    Reading Food Labels ................................................................... 17

    Cooking and Preparation Tips .................................................... 18

Protein Management ............................................................................. 20

Importance of Protein in Kidney Health ............................................. 20

High-Quality Protein Sources ............................................................ 21

Protein Restriction Strategies ............................................................ 22

Adjusting Protein Intake .................................................................... 23

Monitoring Protein Levels ................................................................. 24

Breakfast Recipes ..................................................................................... 25

1. Low-Phosphorus Veggie Omelet .................................................. 25

2. Quinoa Breakfast Bowl ................................................................. 26

3. Low-Protein Banana Pancakes ..................................................... 27

4. Egg White Breakfast Burrito ........................................................ 29

5. Berry and Yogurt Parfait ............................................................... 30

6. Avocado and Tomato Toast .......................................................... 31

7. Cottage Cheese and Pineapple Bowl ........................................... 32

8. Mango and Chia Seed Pudding .................................................... 33

9. Spinach and Feta Breakfast Wrap ................................................ 34

10. Sweet Potato and Turkey Sausage Hash .................................... 35

11. Ricotta and Berry Stuffed French Toast .................................... 36

12. Peanut Butter Banana Smoothie Bowl ....................................... 38

13. Tuna and Cucumber Breakfast Wrap ......................................... 39

14. Chickpea and Spinach Scramble ................................................ 40

15. Coconut and Raspberry Chia Pudding ...................................... 41

16. Tomato and Basil Frittata ..................................................... 42

17. Blueberry Almond Chia Smoothie ..................................... 43

18. Turkey and Veggie Breakfast Skillet ................................... 45

19. Salmon and Asparagus Breakfast Bake ............................... 46

20. Peach and Walnut Breakfast Quinoa .................................. 47

Lunch Recipes ................................................................................ 49

1. Grilled Lemon Herb Chicken ............................................... 49

2. Salmon and Quinoa Salad ..................................................... 50

3. Vegetarian Lentil Soup .......................................................... 51

4. Tofu and Vegetable Stir-Fry .................................................. 53

5. Mediterranean Chickpea Salad .............................................. 54

6. Lemon Dill Shrimp Skewers ................................................. 55

7. Quinoa and Vegetable Stuffed Peppers ................................. 57

8. Chicken and Vegetable Brown Rice Bowl ........................... 58

9. Eggplant and Tomato Ratatouille .......................................... 60

10. Turkey and Spinach Stuffed Mushrooms ............................ 61

11. Cauliflower and Chickpea Curry ......................................... 62

12. Shrimp and Avocado Salad .................................................. 64

13. Spinach and Feta Stuffed Chicken Breast ........................... 65

14. Sweet Potato and Black Bean Bowl .................................... 66

15. Mushroom and Spinach Omelette ....................................... 68

16. Caprese Quinoa Salad ..................................................................69

17. Chicken and Vegetable Skewers ...................................................70

18. Broccoli and Almond Stir-Fry .....................................................71

19. Turkey and Vegetable Wrap .......................................................73

20. Egg Fried Rice with Vegetables .................................................74

Dinner Recipes .......................................................................................76

1. Baked Lemon Herb Tilapia .........................................................76

2. Vegetarian Chickpea and Spinach Curry ....................................77

3. Grilled Rosemary Chicken Breast ..............................................79

4. Mushroom and Spinach Stuffed Bell Peppers ...........................80

5. Baked Garlic and Herb Salmon ..................................................81

6. Quinoa and Black Bean Stuffed Zucchini ..................................83

7. Lemon Garlic Shrimp and Broccoli Stir-Fry ..............................84

8. Eggplant and Tomato Gratin .......................................................85

9. Turkey and Vegetable Skillet ......................................................87

10. Spinach and Feta Stuffed Pork Chops ......................................88

11. Chicken and Vegetable Stir-Fry with Brown Rice ..................89

12. Sesame Ginger Tofu Stir-Fry ....................................................91

13. Spaghetti Squash with Tomato Basil Sauce ............................92

14. Stuffed Portobello Mushrooms with Spinach and Goat Cheese ........................................................................................................94

15. Lemon Herb Grilled Shrimp Skewers ............................. 95

16. Cabbage and Chicken Stir-Fry ..................................... 96

17. Tomato and Basil Baked Chicken Breast ....................... 98

18. Salmon and Asparagus Foil Packets ............................. 99

19. Sesame Orange Glazed Chicken Thighs ..................... 100

20. Vegetable and Shrimp Brown Rice Bowl .................... 102

Dessert Recipes ..................................................................... 104

1. Chia Seed Pudding with Berries ................................... 104

2. Baked Apple with Cinnamon and Walnuts ................... 105

3. Frozen Berry Yogurt Bark ............................................ 106

4. Peach and Almond Sorbet ............................................ 107

5. Vanilla and Berry Parfait ............................................. 108

6. Cinnamon Baked Pears ................................................ 109

7. Avocado Chocolate Mousse ......................................... 110

8. Strawberry Banana Frozen Yogurt ............................... 111

9. Coconut Rice Pudding ................................................. 113

10. Blueberry Almond Oat Bars ....................................... 114

Snack Recipes ........................................................................ 116

1. Cucumber and Hummus Bites ..................................... 116

2. Greek Yogurt and Berry Parfait ................................... 117

3. Rice Cake with Avocado and Cherry Tomatoes ........... 118

4. Apple and Almond Butter Snack ............................................... 119

5. Trail Mix with Nuts and Seeds ................................................. 120

6. Carrot Sticks with Tzatziki Dip ................................................ 121

7. Edamame and Sea Salt Pods .................................................... 122

8. Cottage Cheese and Pineapple Cups ....................................... 123

9. Whole Grain Crackers with Smoked Salmon ......................... 124

10. Banana and Walnut Oat Bites ................................................ 125

28-Day Meal Plan ............................................................................ 127

Conclusion ....................................................................................... 137

# INTRODUCTION

Welcome to the journey of understanding and navigating the intricate landscape of managing Stage 4 Kidney Disease. In this introduction, we'll embark on a conversational exploration, shedding light on the fundamentals of kidney function, the progression that leads to Stage 4, and the pivotal role that diet plays in effectively managing this stage of kidney disease.

Let's start with the basics. Your kidneys are remarkable organs, often described as the body's natural filtration system. They work tirelessly behind the scenes, filtering waste and excess fluids from the blood, producing urine, and maintaining a delicate balance of electrolytes. Picture them as the unsung heroes of your internal health, quietly ensuring the body stays in harmony.

Now, let's delve into the journey to Stage 4 Kidney Disease. This stage represents a significant point in the progression of kidney dysfunction. As the kidneys struggle to perform their vital functions, waste accumulates in the body, leading to a range of complications. Understanding how we arrive at Stage 4 is crucial for grasping the urgency and importance of managing the condition effectively.

Enter the protagonist of our story – diet. It's not just about counting calories or following fads; it's about empowering yourself with the knowledge to make informed choices that directly impact the health of your kidneys. Managing Stage 4 Kidney Disease becomes a delicate dance, and the food you eat is a key partner in this intricate choreography. We'll uncover how specific dietary adjustments can alleviate the burden on your kidneys, promote overall well-being, and potentially slow down the progression of the disease.

So, whether you're here seeking guidance for yourself or supporting a loved one on this journey, buckle up for an enlightening exploration into the world of kidney health, where the choices on your plate can become powerful allies in the battle against Stage 4 Kidney Disease.

# THE BASICS OF A KIDNEY FRIENDLY DIET

## Nutritional Requirements for Stage 4 Kidney Disease

Navigating the dietary landscape with Stage 4 Kidney Disease demands a nuanced understanding of nutritional requirements. At this pivotal stage, the kidneys are less efficient in filtering waste and balancing essential elements in the blood. As a result, tailoring your diet to meet specific nutritional needs becomes paramount.

First and foremost, consider the delicate balance of macronutrients – proteins, fats, and carbohydrates. While proteins are essential for bodily functions, including tissue repair and immune system support, it's crucial to strike a delicate balance. Excessive protein intake can strain the kidneys, contributing to further damage. Collaborate with a healthcare professional or a dietitian to determine your ideal protein intake, considering factors such as age, weight, and overall health.

Beyond proteins, understanding the impact of sodium becomes crucial. Sodium, found abundantly in processed and restaurant-prepared foods, can exacerbate fluid retention and elevate blood pressure. Given the compromised kidney function in Stage 4, adopting a sodium-restricted diet is imperative. Dive into the habit of reading food labels meticulously, opting for fresh, whole foods, and embracing culinary techniques that enhance flavors without relying on excessive salt.

However, it's not just about what to limit but also about what to monitor closely – and that brings us to phosphorus and potassium. Phosphorus, abundant in dairy products, nuts, and seeds, can accumulate in the bloodstream when kidney function is impaired, leading to bone and cardiovascular complications. Likewise, potassium, present in fruits, vegetables, and legumes, needs careful management to prevent imbalances that can impact heart health.

## Protein Intake

In the intricate dance of kidney health, protein intake emerges as a critical partner. Proteins, composed of amino acids, are the building blocks of tissues and play a pivotal role in maintaining the body's structure and function. However, for individuals with Stage 4 Kidney Disease, it's a delicate balancing act.

Understanding the quality of protein is as important as quantity. Opt for high-quality sources like lean meats, fish, eggs, and dairy. These sources provide essential amino acids without the excess burden on compromised kidneys. Consider consulting a dietitian to determine your specific protein needs, aligning them with your overall health goals.

Moreover, consider the concept of "biological value" when evaluating protein sources. Biological value refers to how efficiently the body can use the protein for growth and repair. Animal-based proteins often have a higher biological value compared to plant-based sources, ensuring a more complete and efficient utilization of essential amino acids.

As you embark on this protein-conscious journey, remember that moderation is key. Excessive protein intake can strain the kidneys, leading to a cascade of complications. Adjusting protein intake based on individual needs and periodically reassessing it with healthcare professionals ensures a tailored approach that supports kidney function without undue stress.

## Sodium Restriction

Unlocking the potential of a kidney-friendly diet involves acknowledging the pivotal role of sodium restriction. Sodium, abundant in processed and restaurant-prepared foods, can wreak havoc on individuals with Stage 4 Kidney Disease. Its impact extends beyond mere flavor enhancement; sodium plays a direct role in fluid balance and blood pressure regulation.

Reducing sodium intake is not a one-size-fits-all endeavor; it requires a personalized approach. Collaborate with healthcare professionals or dietitians to establish an optimal sodium limit based on individual health metrics. While general guidelines recommend limiting daily sodium intake to around 2,300 milligrams, individual requirements may vary.

Embracing a sodium-restricted diet involves a paradigm shift in culinary habits. Start by embracing fresh, whole foods and gradually reducing reliance on processed options. Experiment with herbs, spices, and other flavor enhancers that sidestep the need for excessive salt. Remember, it's a gradual process, and taste buds adapt over time to appreciate the natural flavors of food without an overload of sodium.

Understanding hidden sources of sodium is equally crucial. Canned goods, processed meats, and certain condiments can be stealthy contributors to sodium intake. Diligent label reading and a discerning eye for hidden sodium sources empower individuals to make informed choices, mitigating the risk of fluid retention and elevated blood pressure.

## Phosphorus and Potassium Management

The intricacies of a kidney-friendly diet deepen when we turn our attention to phosphorus and potassium management. Both these minerals play vital roles in bodily functions, yet individuals with Stage 4 Kidney Disease must tread carefully to prevent imbalances that could exacerbate their condition.

**Phosphorus**, predominantly found in dairy products, nuts, seeds, and certain grains, poses a unique challenge. In compromised kidney function, the body struggles to excrete excess phosphorus efficiently. This can lead to a buildup in the bloodstream, contributing to bone and cardiovascular issues. Acknowledging the phosphorus content of foods and adopting strategies to limit its absorption become crucial components of dietary management.

Navigating the realm of **potassium management** involves a delicate equilibrium. While potassium is essential for nerve and muscle function, excessive levels can pose risks, especially for individuals with impaired kidneys. Fruits, vegetables, and legumes are rich sources of potassium, and understanding how to balance these in the diet is key.

In this journey, education becomes a powerful tool. Learn to decipher food labels, identifying phosphorus and potassium content. Opt for cooking techniques that leach out excess potassium in certain vegetables. Engage with healthcare professionals or dietitians to create a customized approach, aligning potassium intake with individual health needs.

# SODIUM AND FLUID CONTROL

## Understanding Sodium's Impact

Embarking on a journey to understand sodium's impact on health is like unraveling a hidden narrative within our daily diet. Sodium, an essential mineral, is intricately tied to bodily functions, particularly fluid balance and blood pressure regulation. However, as we delve into the complexities of sodium's role, it becomes evident that moderation and awareness are paramount, especially for individuals navigating Stage 4 Kidney Disease.

Sodium, often associated with its role in enhancing flavor, goes beyond mere taste. It plays a crucial role in maintaining the balance of fluids in and around cells, contributing to nerve function and aiding muscle contractions. In a healthy individual, the kidneys efficiently excrete excess sodium, maintaining a delicate equilibrium. However, with compromised kidney function, this balance becomes precarious.

In the context of Stage 4 Kidney Disease, where the kidneys' ability to filter efficiently is diminished, the impact of sodium magnifies. Excessive sodium intake can lead to fluid retention, edema, and an elevation in blood pressure. This, in turn, places additional strain on the already compromised kidneys, potentially accelerating the progression of kidney disease.

The key to navigating sodium's impact lies in conscious dietary choices. While complete sodium elimination is neither practical nor advisable, moderation becomes the cornerstone. Collaborate with healthcare professionals or dietitians to establish an optimal sodium limit tailored to individual health needs. Adopting a mindful approach to food choices, emphasizing fresh, whole foods, and gradually reducing reliance on processed options, empowers individuals to take control of sodium intake, mitigating its adverse effects.

## Hidden Sodium in Foods

Unraveling the mysteries of sodium control involves peeling back the layers of hidden sodium in foods. While the salt shaker on the dining table is an obvious source, the real challenge lies in identifying and mitigating the concealed sodium present in various processed and restaurant-prepared foods.

Processed foods, often convenient but laden with sodium, pose a significant risk. Canned goods, frozen meals, packaged snacks, and condiments are frequent culprits. The term "sodium-conscious" may be deceptive, as seemingly healthy options may still harbor high sodium content. Vigilance is the key.

Delving into the world of food labels becomes a crucial skill. Sodium hides behind various aliases – sodium chloride, monosodium glutamate (MSG), baking soda, and sodium nitrate, to name a few. Learning to recognize these terms empowers individuals to make informed choices, steering clear of hidden sodium pitfalls.

Restaurant dining introduces another layer of complexity. Dishes prepared outside the home often involve liberal use of salt for flavor enhancement. Understanding how to navigate restaurant menus, communicate dietary needs effectively, and make discerning choices can significantly impact sodium intake. It's not just about what's evident on the plate; it's about uncovering the covert sodium lurking beneath the surface.

## Fluid Intake Guidelines

Fluid intake guidelines take center stage in the intricate dance of sodium and fluid control, particularly for individuals traversing Stage 4 Kidney Disease. While the spotlight often falls on sodium reduction, the symbiotic relationship between sodium and fluid balance necessitates a holistic approach that includes mindful fluid management.

The cornerstone of fluid intake guidelines involves striking a delicate balance. On one hand, adequate hydration is vital for overall health, supporting various bodily functions, including nutrient transportation, temperature regulation, and waste elimination. On the other hand, excessive fluid intake can strain compromised kidneys, leading to fluid retention and elevated blood pressure.

Collaboration with healthcare professionals or dietitians is paramount in establishing personalized fluid intake goals. Factors such as age, weight, climate, and overall health status influence individual hydration needs. Establishing a fluid intake routine that aligns with these factors ensures optimal hydration without overwhelming the kidneys.

Moreover, fluid choices matter. Water, a perennial champion, stands out as the ideal hydrating beverage. Its absence of sodium, calories, and additives makes it a pure and kidney-friendly choice. However, for individuals with specific fluid restrictions, alternatives like herbal teas and diluted fruit juices may be incorporated under professional guidance.

## Balancing Hydration

Balancing hydration is an art, requiring a nuanced understanding of the body's signals and individual health needs. In the realm of Stage 4 Kidney Disease, where fluid balance is intricately linked with sodium control, adopting a mindful and measured approach to hydration is non-negotiable.

Understanding the cues that the body provides is the first step. Thirst, the body's natural indicator, should not be ignored. It's a subtle but powerful signal that prompts us to replenish fluids. However, relying solely on thirst may not be sufficient, especially for individuals with compromised kidney function.

Establishing a structured fluid intake routine can bridge this gap. Distributing fluid intake throughout the day, rather than consuming large amounts at once, helps maintain a steady balance. This approach prevents the kidneys from being overloaded with a sudden influx of fluids, reducing the risk of fluid retention and associated complications.

In the pursuit of balancing hydration, it's essential to recognize that individual needs vary. Factors such as climate, physical activity levels, and overall health status influence the body's demand for fluids. Customizing hydration goals in consultation with healthcare professionals ensures a tailored approach that considers these variables, optimizing hydration without compromising kidney health.

## Monitoring Fluid Levels

The narrative of sodium and fluid control reaches its climax with the crucial act of monitoring fluid levels. This dynamic process involves a keen awareness of individual hydration needs, coupled with an understanding of how the body responds to fluid intake and excretion, particularly in the context of compromised kidney function.

Monitoring fluid levels begins with a partnership with healthcare professionals or dietitians to establish personalized hydration goals. These goals take into account factors such as urine output, weight fluctuations, and overall health status. Regular check-ins and adjustments to fluid intake guidelines ensure a fluid management plan that evolves with the individual's health journey.

Observing urine color and volume becomes a valuable tool in this monitoring process. Light yellow urine generally indicates adequate hydration, while dark yellow or amber tones may signal dehydration. However, it's important to note that certain medications or supplements can influence urine color, emphasizing the need for a holistic approach to fluid level assessment.

Weight monitoring also plays a pivotal role. Sudden or significant fluctuations in weight may indicate fluid retention, necessitating adjustments to fluid intake. However, it's crucial to distinguish between fat and fluid changes, requiring a nuanced understanding that healthcare professionals can provide.

In the grand finale of sodium and fluid control, the act of monitoring becomes a constant dialogue between the individual and their healthcare team. It's a journey of self-awareness, where the body's signals and responses are decoded in collaboration with professionals who provide guidance, support, and adjustments to fluid management strategies.

# MANAGING PHOSPHORUS AND POTASSIUM

## Impact of Phosphorus and Potassium on Kidney Health

Embarking on the journey of managing Stage 4 Kidney Disease unveils a chapter marked by the nuanced control of phosphorus and potassium. These two minerals, essential for various bodily functions, take center stage in the intricate dance of kidney health. Understanding their impact on compromised kidneys becomes crucial in crafting a dietary strategy that not only addresses nutritional needs but also safeguards against potential complications.

**Phosphorus**, a mineral abundantly present in foods, plays a pivotal role in bone health, energy metabolism, and acid-base balance within the body. However, when kidney function is compromised, the body's ability to regulate phosphorus levels diminishes. This can lead to a buildup of phosphorus in the bloodstream, contributing to bone and cardiovascular issues. Recognizing the impact of phosphorus on kidney health sets the stage for informed dietary choices and proactive management.

Similarly, **potassium**, another essential mineral, is integral to nerve and muscle function, maintaining heart rhythm, and balancing bodily fluids. While potassium is crucial for overall health, excessive levels can pose risks, particularly for individuals with impaired kidneys. Managing potassium becomes a delicate balancing act to prevent imbalances that could exacerbate kidney-related complications.

In the realm of Stage 4 Kidney Disease, the impact of phosphorus and potassium extends beyond mere nutritional considerations. It becomes a strategic approach to support kidney function, mitigate potential risks, and foster overall well-being.

## Phosphorus-Rich Foods

Understanding the landscape of phosphorus-rich foods is the first step in the meticulous management of Stage 4 Kidney Disease. Phosphorus lurks in various dietary sources, both plant and animal-based, making it imperative for individuals to discern and control their phosphorus intake.

Animal products, including dairy, meat, and poultry, are primary contributors to dietary phosphorus. Dairy, often lauded for its bone-strengthening properties, paradoxically becomes a potential source of excess phosphorus for individuals with compromised kidneys. Understanding how to balance dairy consumption to meet nutritional needs without overwhelming phosphorus levels becomes crucial.

On the plant-based front, nuts, seeds, legumes, and whole grains also harbor phosphorus. While these foods are nutritionally dense and offer various health benefits, they require a measured approach in the context of Stage 4 Kidney Disease. Strategically incorporating these foods into the diet, coupled with monitoring overall phosphorus intake, allows for a nuanced dietary strategy that supports kidney health.

The challenge lies not in complete phosphorus elimination but in informed choices that align with individual health needs. Collaborating with healthcare professionals or dietitians to establish personalized phosphorus goals ensures a tailored approach that considers nutritional requirements while mitigating potential risks.

## Potassium-Rich Foods

Potassium-rich foods, celebrated for their role in supporting various bodily functions, present a dual challenge for individuals managing Stage 4 Kidney Disease. On one hand, potassium is essential; on the other, excessive intake can pose risks. Navigating this delicate balance involves a comprehensive understanding of potassium-rich foods and strategic dietary choices.

Fruits and vegetables, touted for their nutritional prowess, are primary sources of potassium. Bananas, oranges, potatoes, tomatoes, and leafy greens are among the potassium-rich culprits. While these foods offer an array of health benefits, their integration into the diet demands thoughtful consideration in the context of compromised kidney function.

Understanding the concept of portion control becomes paramount. Consuming smaller portions of potassium-rich foods throughout the day, rather than in concentrated amounts, allows for a more gradual and manageable intake. This measured approach reduces the risk of potassium spikes that could potentially impact heart health.

Cooking methods also play a role in managing potassium. Certain techniques, such as boiling or soaking vegetables, can leach out potassium, making them more kidney-friendly. The integration of these culinary strategies empowers individuals to savor the nutritional benefits of potassium-rich foods without compromising kidney health.

As with phosphorus, collaboration with healthcare professionals or dietitians is key. Establishing personalized potassium goals, aligning them with individual health metrics, and periodically reassessing dietary strategies ensure a balanced and tailored approach to potassium management.

## Strategies for Phosphorus and Potassium Control

The crux of effective management lies in the development and implementation of strategies for phosphorus and potassium control. It's not about restriction but rather about conscious choices, informed decision-making, and a proactive approach that considers individual health needs.

## Reading Food Labels

In the labyrinth of food choices, the ability to decipher and interpret food labels emerges as a powerful tool. Food labels provide a roadmap, offering insights into the nutritional content of packaged products. For individuals managing Stage 4 Kidney Disease, mastering the art of reading food labels becomes an essential skill in the journey of phosphorus and potassium control.

Focus on the phosphorus and potassium content listed on labels, paying attention to both absolute values and serving sizes. Sodium phosphate, a common additive, is a source of hidden phosphorus, while potassium-based additives can contribute to potassium intake. Recognizing these ingredients empowers individuals to make conscious choices, avoiding potential pitfalls in their quest for a kidney-friendly diet.

Understand that terms like "low phosphorus" or "low potassium" on labels may not universally apply. Individual dietary goals and restrictions vary, necessitating a personalized approach. Collaborate with healthcare professionals or dietitians to establish specific benchmarks tailored to individual health needs.

## Cooking and Preparation Tips

The kitchen transforms into a battleground for phosphorus and potassium control, where culinary choices become strategic maneuvers in the pursuit of a kidney-friendly diet. Embracing cooking and preparation tips that mitigate phosphorus and potassium content while preserving nutritional value allows for a harmonious fusion of health-conscious and flavorful dining.

Consider adopting cooking techniques that reduce phosphorus and potassium levels in foods. Soaking beans and legumes before cooking, choosing fresh over processed meats, and using certain cooking methods that leach out these minerals contribute to a kidney-friendly culinary landscape.

Experiment with herbs, spices, and alternative flavor enhancers to reduce reliance on salt, which might be restricted for sodium control. This not only adds depth to the culinary experience but also aligns with the broader goal of maintaining a well-rounded and enjoyable diet.

The integration of phosphorus and potassium control into cooking extends beyond individual meal preparation to encompass overall meal planning. Collaborate with healthcare professionals or dietitians to craft well-balanced meal plans that consider both nutritional requirements and the need for phosphorus and potassium control. This ensures a holistic approach to dietary management that supports kidney health without compromising on culinary enjoyment.

In the intricate tapestry of phosphorus and potassium management, reading food labels and embracing cooking and preparation tips emerge as pillars of empowerment. These strategies, when combined with a nuanced understanding of phosphorus and potassium-rich foods, offer individuals navigating Stage 4 Kidney Disease the tools to make informed choices, cultivate a kidney-friendly diet, and foster overall well-being.

# PROTEIN MANAGEMENT

## Importance of Protein in Kidney Health

Protein, the cornerstone of tissue repair, immune function, and overall vitality, plays a crucial role in maintaining optimal health. However, for individuals navigating Stage 4 Kidney Disease, the significance of protein takes center stage in a delicate balancing act. Understanding the intricate relationship between protein and kidney health is fundamental to crafting a dietary approach that supports overall well-being.

Proteins are composed of amino acids, often referred to as the building blocks of life. These amino acids are essential for the synthesis of enzymes, hormones, and structural components of tissues. In the context of kidney health, protein plays a pivotal role in preserving muscle mass, a concern for individuals facing the challenges of Stage 4 Kidney Disease.

While protein is undeniably essential, the compromised filtration capacity of the kidneys at this stage necessitates a thoughtful and strategic approach. Excessive protein intake can burden the kidneys, contributing to the progression of kidney disease. Striking the right balance, therefore, becomes crucial, and this balance is achievable through an understanding of high-quality protein sources, protein restriction strategies, and personalized adjustments to protein intake.

# High-Quality Protein Sources

The journey of protein management begins with the exploration of high-quality protein sources that not only meet nutritional needs but also align with the demands of compromised kidney function. Opting for proteins that provide a complete array of essential amino acids without overburdening the kidneys becomes a guiding principle.

Animal-based proteins, such as lean meats, poultry, fish, eggs, and dairy, stand out as exemplary sources of high-quality protein. These sources offer a robust profile of essential amino acids, ensuring the body receives the necessary building blocks for optimal functioning. Incorporating these proteins into the diet supports muscle maintenance and overall health.

For those inclined towards plant-based options, legumes, tofu, and certain grains can contribute valuable protein without the same burden on the kidneys. Combining various plant-based protein sources can create a complementary amino acid profile, enhancing the overall nutritional value of the diet.

Navigating high-quality protein sources involves a nuanced understanding of individual preferences, dietary restrictions, and health goals. Collaborating with healthcare professionals or dietitians allows for the customization of protein choices based on individual needs, creating a balanced and kidney-friendly approach to nutrition.

# Protein Restriction Strategies

Recognizing the importance of protein in kidney health doesn't negate the need for strategic protein restriction in the context of Stage 4 Kidney Disease. Protein restriction strategies aim to optimize protein intake, mitigating the strain on compromised kidneys while ensuring adequate nutritional support.

One approach to protein restriction involves controlling the total amount of protein consumed daily. Collaborating with healthcare professionals or dietitians allows individuals to establish personalized protein goals tailored to their specific health metrics. These goals consider factors such as age, weight, and overall health status, ensuring a targeted and individualized strategy.

Another facet of protein restriction involves managing the type of protein consumed. While animal-based proteins offer a complete array of essential amino acids, their higher phosphorus content can pose challenges for individuals with kidney disease. Adjusting the balance between animal and plant-based proteins, under professional guidance, allows for a nuanced approach that addresses nutritional needs while managing phosphorus levels.

It's essential to note that protein restriction strategies are not about deprivation but rather about optimization. They are a proactive measure to preserve kidney function, support overall health, and create a sustainable dietary approach that aligns with individual well-being.

# Adjusting Protein Intake

The journey of protein management in Stage 4 Kidney Disease involves a dynamic process of adjusting protein intake based on evolving health needs, lifestyle changes, and overall well-being. Recognizing that protein requirements may fluctuate over time, especially in response to health status, prompts the need for a flexible and personalized approach.

Adjusting protein intake is not a one-size-fits-all endeavor. Life circumstances, health conditions, and treatment plans can influence protein needs. Periodic assessments, conducted in collaboration with healthcare professionals or dietitians, allow for adjustments to protein goals, ensuring they align with the individual's health journey.

Life events such as surgery, illness, or changes in physical activity levels may necessitate temporary modifications to protein intake. In such instances, proactive communication with healthcare providers ensures that dietary adjustments are supportive rather than detrimental to overall health.

Moreover, adjusting protein intake involves considering the broader nutritional landscape. Collaborating with healthcare professionals allows for the integration of protein adjustments within a comprehensive dietary strategy that supports overall health, addresses nutrient needs, and fosters an environment conducive to kidney well-being.

# Monitoring Protein Levels

The final act in the symphony of protein management is the vigilant monitoring of protein levels. This involves a dynamic dialogue between the individual and their healthcare team, where regular assessments and adjustments ensure that protein intake remains in harmony with kidney health.

Monitoring protein levels requires routine check-ins with healthcare professionals or dietitians to assess the impact of dietary choices on kidney function. Laboratory tests, including blood urea nitrogen (BUN) and serum creatinine, provide valuable insights into how the kidneys are responding to protein intake. Regular monitoring allows for the early identification of trends or deviations, enabling timely adjustments to dietary strategies.

Beyond numerical indicators, paying attention to physical cues and overall well-being forms an integral part of monitoring protein levels. Individual responses to dietary changes, energy levels, and muscle mass maintenance offer valuable qualitative insights. This holistic approach ensures that protein management aligns not only with laboratory values but also with the individual's overall health goals and quality of life.

# BREAKFAST RECIPES

## 1. Low-Phosphorus Veggie Omelet

**Prep Time:** 10 minutes
**Cooking Time:** 10 minutes
**Serving Size:** 1

**Ingredients:**

- 2 large eggs
- 1/4 cup bell peppers, diced
- 1/4 cup spinach, chopped
- 1/4 cup mushrooms, sliced
- 1 tablespoon olive oil
- Salt and pepper to taste

**Instructions:**

1. In a bowl, whisk eggs until well-beaten.
2. Heat olive oil in a non-stick skillet over medium heat.
3. Add bell peppers, spinach, and mushrooms to the skillet. Sauté until vegetables are tender.
4. Pour beaten eggs over the vegetables, allowing them to set for a moment.

5. Gently lift the edges of the omelet to allow uncooked eggs to flow underneath.

6. Once the eggs are mostly set, fold the omelet in half.

7. Cook for an additional 2-3 minutes until fully cooked.

8. Season with salt and pepper to taste.

**Nutritional Information (per serving):**

- Calories: 220
- Protein: 15g
- Phosphorus: 150mg
- Potassium: 250mg

# 2. Quinoa Breakfast Bowl

**Prep Time:** 15 minutes
**Cooking Time:** 15 minutes
**Serving Size:** 1

**Ingredients:**

- 1/2 cup cooked quinoa
- 1/4 cup blueberries
- 1/4 cup sliced strawberries
- 1 tablespoon chopped almonds

- 1 tablespoon honey
- 1/2 teaspoon cinnamon

**Instructions:**

1. In a bowl, combine cooked quinoa, blueberries, strawberries, and chopped almonds.
2. Drizzle honey over the mixture.
3. Sprinkle cinnamon on top.
4. Mix well and enjoy.

**Nutritional Information (per serving):**

- Calories: 280
- Protein: 10g
- Phosphorus: 120mg
- Potassium: 180mg

# 3. Low-Protein Banana Pancakes

**Prep Time:** 15 minutes
**Cooking Time:** 10 minutes
**Serving Size:** 2 pancakes

**Ingredients:**

- 1 ripe banana, mashed

- 1/2 cup oat flour
- 1/4 cup almond milk
- 1/2 teaspoon baking powder
- 1/4 teaspoon cinnamon
- 1 tablespoon coconut oil

**Instructions:**

1. In a bowl, mix mashed banana, oat flour, almond milk, baking powder, and cinnamon.
2. Heat coconut oil in a skillet over medium heat.
3. Spoon batter onto the skillet to form pancakes.
4. Cook until bubbles appear on the surface, then flip and cook the other side.
5. Serve with fresh berries or a drizzle of honey.

**Nutritional Information (per serving - 2 pancakes):**

- Calories: 300
- Protein: 6g
- Phosphorus: 80mg
- Potassium: 180mg

# 4. Egg White Breakfast Burrito

**Prep Time:** 15 minutes

**Cooking Time:** 10 minutes

**Serving Size:** 1

**Ingredients:**

- 2 large egg whites
- 1/4 cup black beans, drained and rinsed
- 2 tablespoons salsa
- 1 tablespoon diced avocado
- 1 whole-grain tortilla

**Instructions:**

1. Whisk egg whites in a bowl until frothy.
2. Cook egg whites in a non-stick skillet over medium heat.
3. Warm the tortilla in the skillet or microwave.
4. Fill the tortilla with cooked egg whites, black beans, salsa, and diced avocado.
5. Fold the sides of the tortilla to form a burrito.

**Nutritional Information (per serving):**

- Calories: 250
- Protein: 18g

- Phosphorus: 100mg
- Potassium: 200mg

## 5. Berry and Yogurt Parfait

**Prep Time:** 10 minutes
**Serving Size:** 1

**Ingredients:**

- 1/2 cup low-fat Greek yogurt
- 1/4 cup granola (low-phosphorus)
- 1/4 cup mixed berries (blueberries, strawberries)
- 1 tablespoon honey

**Instructions:**

1. In a glass or bowl, layer Greek yogurt, granola, and mixed berries.
2. Drizzle honey on top.
3. Repeat the layers.
4. Garnish with a few fresh berries on the top.

**Nutritional Information (per serving):**

- Calories: 280
- Protein: 15g

- Phosphorus: 100mg
- Potassium: 150mg

## 6. Avocado and Tomato Toast

**Prep Time:** 10 minutes
**Cooking Time:** 5 minutes
**Serving Size:** 1

**Ingredients:**

- 1 slice whole-grain bread
- 1/2 avocado, mashed
- 1/2 cup cherry tomatoes, halved
- 1 teaspoon olive oil
- Salt and pepper to taste

**Instructions:**

1. Toast the whole-grain bread slice.
2. Spread mashed avocado on the toast.
3. Arrange halved cherry tomatoes on top.
4. Drizzle olive oil and season with salt and pepper.

**Nutritional Information (per serving):**

- Calories: 230

- Protein: 5g

- Phosphorus: 90mg

- Potassium: 300mg

## 7. Cottage Cheese and Pineapple Bowl

**Prep Time:** 10 minutes
**Serving Size:** 1

**Ingredients:**

- 1/2 cup low-fat cottage cheese

- 1/2 cup fresh pineapple chunks

- 1 tablespoon chopped walnuts

- 1 teaspoon honey

**Instructions:**

1. In a bowl, combine cottage cheese and fresh pineapple chunks.

2. Sprinkle chopped walnuts on top.

3. Drizzle honey over the mixture.

**Nutritional Information (per serving):**

- Calories: 280

- Protein: 15g

- Phosphorus: 120mg
- Potassium: 200mg

## 8. Mango and Chia Seed Pudding

**Prep Time:** 10 minutes (+ overnight chilling)
**Serving Size:** 1

**Ingredients:**

- 1/4 cup chia seeds
- 1 cup almond milk
- 1/2 mango, diced
- 1 tablespoon unsweetened shredded coconut

**Instructions:**

1. In a jar, mix chia seeds and almond milk. Stir well.
2. Refrigerate overnight or for at least 4 hours.
3. In the morning, layer chia pudding with diced mango.
4. Sprinkle unsweetened shredded coconut on top.

**Nutritional Information (per serving):**

- Calories: 290
- Protein: 8g

- Phosphorus: 80mg
- Potassium: 180mg

## 9. Spinach and Feta Breakfast Wrap

**Prep Time:** 15 minutes
**Cooking Time:** 5 minutes
**Serving Size:** 1

**Ingredients:**

- 1 whole-grain tortilla
- 2 large eggs, scrambled
- 1/2 cup fresh spinach
- 2 tablespoons crumbled feta cheese
- 1/4 cup cherry tomatoes, sliced

**Instructions:**

1. Cook scrambled eggs in a non-stick skillet.
2. Warm the tortilla in the skillet or microwave.
3. Layer the tortilla with fresh spinach, scrambled eggs, crumbled feta, and sliced cherry tomatoes.
4. Roll the tortilla to form a wrap.

**Nutritional Information (per serving):**

- Calories: 320
- Protein: 18g
- Phosphorus: 120mg
- Potassium: 250mg

## 10. Sweet Potato and Turkey Sausage Hash

**Prep Time:** 20 minutes
**Cooking Time:** 15 minutes
**Serving Size:** 1

**Ingredients:**

- 1 small sweet potato, diced
- 2 turkey sausage links, sliced
- 1/4 cup red bell pepper, diced
- 1/4 cup yellow onion, diced
- 1 tablespoon olive oil
- 1/2 teaspoon paprika
- Salt and pepper to taste

**Instructions:**

1. In a skillet, heat olive oil over medium heat.

2. Add diced sweet potato, turkey sausage, red bell pepper, and onion.

3. Cook until sweet potatoes are tender and sausage is browned.

4. Sprinkle with paprika, salt, and pepper to taste.

**Nutritional Information (per serving):**

- Calories: 330
- Protein: 15g
- Phosphorus: 150mg
- Potassium: 350mg

## 11. Ricotta and Berry Stuffed French Toast

**Prep Time:** 15 minutes
**Cooking Time:** 10 minutes
**Serving Size:** 1

**Ingredients:**

- 2 slices whole-grain bread
- 1/4 cup low-fat ricotta cheese
- 1/4 cup mixed berries (blueberries, strawberries)
- 1 large egg
- 1/4 cup almond milk

- 1/2 teaspoon vanilla extract
- 1 teaspoon maple syrup (optional)

**Instructions:**

1. In a bowl, mix ricotta cheese and mixed berries.
2. Spread the mixture on one slice of bread and top with the other slice, creating a sandwich.
3. In another bowl, whisk together egg, almond milk, and vanilla extract.
4. Dip the sandwich into the egg mixture, ensuring both sides are coated.
5. Cook in a skillet over medium heat until both sides are golden brown.
6. Drizzle with maple syrup if desired.

**Nutritional Information (per serving):**

- Calories: 350
- Protein: 15g
- Phosphorus: 120mg
- Potassium: 200mg

# 12. Peanut Butter Banana Smoothie Bowl

**Prep Time:** 10 minutes

**Serving Size:** 1

**Ingredients:**

- 1 frozen banana
- 1/2 cup unsweetened almond milk
- 1 tablespoon peanut butter
- 1 tablespoon chia seeds
- Toppings: sliced banana, granola, and a drizzle of honey

**Instructions:**

1. In a blender, combine frozen banana, almond milk, peanut butter, and chia seeds.
2. Blend until smooth.
3. Pour the smoothie into a bowl.
4. Top with sliced banana, granola, and a drizzle of honey.

**Nutritional Information (per serving):**

- Calories: 320
- Protein: 8g
- Phosphorus: 90mg
- Potassium: 350mg

## 13. Tuna and Cucumber Breakfast Wrap

**Prep Time:** 10 minutes

**Serving Size:** 1

**Ingredients:**

- 1 whole-grain tortilla
- 1/2 can tuna, drained
- 1/4 cup cucumber, sliced
- 1 tablespoon plain Greek yogurt
- 1/2 teaspoon dill
- Salt and pepper to taste

**Instructions:**

1. In a bowl, mix tuna, sliced cucumber, Greek yogurt, dill, salt, and pepper.
2. Warm the tortilla in the skillet or microwave.
3. Spread the tuna mixture on the tortilla.
4. Roll the tortilla to form a wrap.

**Nutritional Information (per serving):**

- Calories: 280
- Protein: 20g
- Phosphorus: 150mg

- Potassium: 200mg

## 14. Chickpea and Spinach Scramble

**Prep Time:** 15 minutes
**Cooking Time:** 10 minutes
**Serving Size:** 1

**Ingredients:**

- 1/2 cup canned chickpeas, drained
- 2 large eggs, scrambled
- 1/4 cup spinach, chopped
- 1/4 cup cherry tomatoes, halved
- 1 tablespoon feta cheese, crumbled
- 1 teaspoon olive oil
- Salt and pepper to taste

**Instructions:**

1. In a skillet, heat olive oil over medium heat.
2. Add chickpeas, spinach, and cherry tomatoes. Sauté until spinach wilts.
3. Add scrambled eggs and cook until fully cooked.
4. Sprinkle crumbled feta on top.

5. Season with salt and pepper to taste.

**Nutritional Information (per serving):**

- Calories: 310
- Protein: 18g
- Phosphorus: 120mg
- Potassium: 250mg

## 15. Coconut and Raspberry Chia Pudding

**Prep Time:** 10 minutes (+ overnight chilling)

**Serving Size:** 1

**Ingredients:**

- 1/4 cup chia seeds
- 1 cup coconut milk
- 1/4 cup fresh raspberries
- 1 tablespoon shredded coconut

**Instructions:**

1. In a jar, mix chia seeds and coconut milk. Stir well.
2. Refrigerate overnight or for at least 4 hours.
3. In the morning, layer chia pudding with fresh raspberries.

4. Sprinkle shredded coconut on top.

**Nutritional Information (per serving):**

- Calories: 290
- Protein: 6g
- Phosphorus: 80mg
- Potassium: 180mg

## 16. Tomato and Basil Frittata

**Prep Time:** 15 minutes
**Cooking Time:** 15 minutes
**Serving Size:** 1

**Ingredients:**

- 2 large eggs
- 1/4 cup cherry tomatoes, halved
- 1 tablespoon fresh basil, chopped
- 1 tablespoon Parmesan cheese, grated
- 1 teaspoon olive oil
- Salt and pepper to taste

**Instructions:**

1. Preheat the oven broiler.

2. In a bowl, whisk eggs until well-beaten.

3. Heat olive oil in an oven-safe skillet over medium heat.

4. Add cherry tomatoes and cook until they start to soften.

5. Pour beaten eggs over the tomatoes.

6. Sprinkle fresh basil and grated Parmesan on top.

7. Transfer the skillet to the oven and broil until the frittata is set and lightly browned.

8. Season with salt and pepper to taste.

**Nutritional Information (per serving):**

- Calories: 250
- Protein: 14g
- Phosphorus: 130mg
- Potassium: 200mg

## 17. Blueberry Almond Chia Smoothie

**Prep Time:** 10 minutes
**Serving Size:** 1

**Ingredients:**

- 1/2 cup blueberries (fresh or frozen)
- 1/2 banana

- 1 tablespoon almond butter
- 1 tablespoon chia seeds
- 1/2 cup unsweetened almond milk
- Ice cubes (optional)

**Instructions:**

1. In a blender, combine blueberries, banana, almond butter, chia seeds, and almond milk.
2. Blend until smooth.
3. Add ice cubes if desired and blend again.

**Nutritional Information (per serving):**

- Calories: 280
- Protein: 8g
- Phosphorus: 90mg
- Potassium: 220mg

## 18. Turkey and Veggie Breakfast Skillet

**Prep Time:** 15 minutes
**Cooking Time:** 15 minutes
**Serving Size:** 1

**Ingredients:**

- 1/2 cup lean ground turkey
- 1/4 cup zucchini, diced
- 1/4 cup red bell pepper, diced
- 2 large eggs
- 1 tablespoon olive oil
- 1/2 teaspoon cumin
- Salt and pepper to taste

**Instructions:**

1. In a skillet, heat olive oil over medium heat.
2. Add ground turkey and cook until browned.
3. Add diced zucchini and red bell pepper. Sauté until vegetables are tender.
4. Sprinkle cumin, salt, and pepper.
5. Create wells in the skillet and crack eggs into them.
6. Cover and cook until the eggs are cooked to your liking.

**Nutritional Information (per serving):**

- Calories: 330
- Protein: 24g
- Phosphorus: 180mg
- Potassium: 250mg

## 19. Salmon and Asparagus Breakfast Bake

**Prep Time:** 20 minutes
**Cooking Time:** 20 minutes
**Serving Size:** 1

**Ingredients:**

- 4 ounces salmon fillet
- 1/2 cup asparagus, chopped
- 2 large eggs
- 1 tablespoon dill, chopped
- 1 teaspoon olive oil
- Salt and pepper to taste

**Instructions:**

1. Preheat the oven to 375°F (190°C).
2. Place salmon and chopped asparagus on a baking sheet.

3. Drizzle with olive oil and sprinkle with salt, pepper, and chopped dill.

4. Bake for 15-20 minutes until the salmon is cooked through.

5. In a separate skillet, cook eggs to your liking.

6. Serve the baked salmon and asparagus with the eggs on top.

**Nutritional Information (per serving):**

- Calories: 350
- Protein: 30g
- Phosphorus: 200mg
- Potassium: 350mg

## 20. Peach and Walnut Breakfast Quinoa

**Prep Time:** 15 minutes
**Cooking Time:** 15 minutes
**Serving Size:** 1

**Ingredients:**

- 1/2 cup cooked quinoa
- 1 peach, diced
- 1 tablespoon chopped walnuts
- 1 tablespoon honey

- 1/2 teaspoon cinnamon

**Instructions:**

1. In a bowl, combine cooked quinoa, diced peach, and chopped walnuts.

2. Drizzle honey over the mixture.

3. Sprinkle cinnamon on top.

4. Mix well and enjoy.

**Nutritional Information (per serving):**

- Calories: 300
- Protein: 8g
- Phosphorus: 120mg
- Potassium: 200mg

# LUNCH RECIPES

## 1. Grilled Lemon Herb Chicken

**Prep Time:** 10 minutes
**Cooking Time:** 15 minutes
**Serving Size:** 1

**Ingredients:**

- 4 ounces boneless, skinless chicken breast
- 1 tablespoon olive oil
- 1 teaspoon lemon zest
- 1 tablespoon fresh lemon juice
- 1 teaspoon dried oregano
- Salt and pepper to taste

**Instructions:**

1. Preheat the grill to medium-high heat.
2. In a bowl, mix olive oil, lemon zest, lemon juice, oregano, salt, and pepper.
3. Brush the chicken breast with the mixture.
4. Grill the chicken for about 7-8 minutes per side or until fully cooked.

5. Let it rest for a few minutes before serving.

**Nutritional Information (per serving):**

- Calories: 250
- Protein: 30g
- Phosphorus: 180mg
- Potassium: 280mg

# 2. Salmon and Quinoa Salad

**Prep Time:** 15 minutes
**Cooking Time:** 15 minutes
**Serving Size:** 1

**Ingredients:**

- 4 ounces salmon fillet
- 1/2 cup cooked quinoa
- 1 cup mixed greens
- 1/4 cup cherry tomatoes, halved
- 1/4 cup cucumber, sliced
- 1 tablespoon olive oil
- 1 tablespoon balsamic vinegar
- Salt and pepper to taste

**Instructions:**

1. Season salmon with salt and pepper, then bake or grill until cooked.
2. In a bowl, mix cooked quinoa, mixed greens, cherry tomatoes, and cucumber.
3. Place the cooked salmon on top.
4. Drizzle with olive oil and balsamic vinegar.

**Nutritional Information (per serving):**

- Calories: 320
- Protein: 25g
- Phosphorus: 200mg
- Potassium: 350mg

# 3. Vegetarian Lentil Soup

**Prep Time:** 15 minutes
**Cooking Time:** 30 minutes
**Serving Size:** 1

**Ingredients:**

- 1/2 cup dry lentils, rinsed and drained
- 1/4 cup onion, chopped

- 1/4 cup carrot, diced
- 1/4 cup celery, chopped
- 2 cups low-sodium vegetable broth
- 1 teaspoon olive oil
- 1/2 teaspoon cumin
- 1/2 teaspoon turmeric
- Salt and pepper to taste

**Instructions:**

1. In a pot, heat olive oil over medium heat.
2. Add chopped onion, carrot, and celery. Sauté until softened.
3. Add lentils, vegetable broth, cumin, turmeric, salt, and pepper.
4. Bring to a boil, then reduce heat and simmer for 25-30 minutes until lentils are tender.

**Nutritional Information (per serving):**

- Calories: 280
- Protein: 18g
- Phosphorus: 150mg
- Potassium: 400mg

# 4. Tofu and Vegetable Stir-Fry

**Prep Time:** 20 minutes
**Cooking Time:** 15 minutes
**Serving Size:** 1

**Ingredients:**

- 1/2 cup firm tofu, cubed
- 1/2 cup broccoli florets
- 1/4 cup bell peppers, sliced
- 1/4 cup snap peas
- 1 tablespoon low-sodium soy sauce
- 1 tablespoon sesame oil
- 1 teaspoon ginger, minced
- 1 clove garlic, minced

**Instructions:**

1. In a wok or skillet, heat sesame oil over medium-high heat.
2. Add cubed tofu and stir-fry until golden brown.
3. Add broccoli, bell peppers, snap peas, ginger, and garlic. Stir-fry for 5-7 minutes.
4. Pour in soy sauce and continue cooking until vegetables are tender.

**Nutritional Information (per serving):**

- Calories: 290
- Protein: 20g
- Phosphorus: 200mg
- Potassium: 350mg

## 5. Mediterranean Chickpea Salad

**Prep Time:** 15 minutes
**Serving Size:** 1

**Ingredients:**

- 1/2 cup canned chickpeas, drained and rinsed
- 1/4 cup cherry tomatoes, halved
- 1/4 cup cucumber, diced
- 1/4 cup feta cheese, crumbled
- 1 tablespoon Kalamata olives, sliced
- 1 tablespoon olive oil
- 1 tablespoon red wine vinegar
- 1 teaspoon dried oregano
- Salt and pepper to taste

**Instructions:**

1. In a bowl, combine chickpeas, cherry tomatoes, cucumber, feta cheese, and olives.

2. In a small bowl, whisk together olive oil, red wine vinegar, oregano, salt, and pepper.

3. Pour the dressing over the salad and toss gently.

**Nutritional Information (per serving):**

- Calories: 320
- Protein: 15g
- Phosphorus: 180mg
- Potassium: 250mg

## 6. Lemon Dill Shrimp Skewers

**Prep Time:** 15 minutes
**Cooking Time:** 10 minutes
**Serving Size:** 1

**Ingredients:**

- 4 ounces shrimp, peeled and deveined
- 1 tablespoon olive oil
- 1 teaspoon lemon zest

- 1 tablespoon fresh lemon juice
- 1 teaspoon fresh dill, chopped
- Salt and pepper to taste

**Instructions:**

1. Preheat the grill or broiler.
2. In a bowl, mix olive oil, lemon zest, lemon juice, chopped dill, salt, and pepper.
3. Thread shrimp onto skewers and brush with the lemon mixture.
4. Grill or broil for 3-4 minutes per side until shrimp are opaque.

**Nutritional Information (per serving):**

- Calories: 220
- Protein: 25g
- Phosphorus: 200mg
- Potassium: 180mg

# 7. Quinoa and Vegetable Stuffed Peppers

**Prep Time:** 20 minutes
**Cooking Time:** 25 minutes
**Serving Size:** 1

**Ingredients:**

- 1/2 cup cooked quinoa
- 2 bell peppers, halved and seeds removed
- 1/4 cup black beans, drained and rinsed
- 1/4 cup corn kernels
- 1/4 cup diced tomatoes
- 1/4 cup diced red onion
- 1/4 cup shredded low-phosphorus cheese
- 1 tablespoon olive oil
- 1 teaspoon cumin
- Salt and pepper to taste

**Instructions:**

1. Preheat the oven to 375°F (190°C).
2. In a bowl, mix cooked quinoa, black beans, corn, tomatoes, red onion, cheese, olive oil, cumin, salt, and pepper.
3. Stuff the halved bell peppers with the quinoa mixture.

4. Bake for 20-25 minutes until peppers are tender.

**Nutritional Information (per serving):**

- Calories: 310
- Protein: 15g
- Phosphorus: 180mg
- Potassium: 350mg

# 8. Chicken and Vegetable Brown Rice Bowl

**Prep Time:** 15 minutes
**Cooking Time:** 20 minutes
**Serving Size:** 1

**Ingredients:**

- 4 ounces boneless, skinless chicken breast, diced
- 1/2 cup cooked brown rice
- 1/4 cup broccoli florets
- 1/4 cup carrots, sliced
- 1/4 cup snow peas
- 1 tablespoon low-sodium soy sauce
- 1 teaspoon sesame oil
- 1 teaspoon ginger, minced

- 1 clove garlic, minced

**Instructions:**

1. In a wok or skillet, heat sesame oil over medium-high heat.

2. Add diced chicken and cook until browned.

3. Add broccoli, carrots, snow peas, ginger, and garlic. Stir-fry for 5-7 minutes.

4. Pour in soy sauce and continue cooking until vegetables are tender.

5. Serve over cooked brown rice.

**Nutritional Information (per serving):**

- Calories: 320

- Protein: 25g

- Phosphorus: 200mg

- Potassium: 350mg

## 9. Eggplant and Tomato Ratatouille

**Prep Time:** 20 minutes
**Cooking Time:** 25 minutes
**Serving Size:** 1

**Ingredients:**

- 1/2 cup eggplant, diced
- 1/4 cup zucchini, sliced
- 1/4 cup bell peppers, diced
- 1/4 cup tomatoes, diced
- 2 tablespoons olive oil
- 1 teaspoon dried thyme
- 1 teaspoon dried rosemary
- Salt and pepper to taste

**Instructions:**

1. Preheat the oven to 375°F (190°C).
2. In a baking dish, combine diced eggplant, sliced zucchini, diced bell peppers, and tomatoes.
3. Drizzle with olive oil and sprinkle with thyme, rosemary, salt, and pepper.
4. Toss to coat vegetables evenly.

5. Bake for 20-25 minutes until vegetables are tender.

**Nutritional Information (per serving):**

- Calories: 280
- Protein: 10g
- Phosphorus: 120mg
- Potassium: 400mg

## 10. Turkey and Spinach Stuffed Mushrooms

**Prep Time:** 20 minutes
**Cooking Time:** 15 minutes
**Serving Size:** 1

**Ingredients:**

- 4 large mushrooms, stems removed
- 1/2 cup lean ground turkey
- 1/4 cup spinach, chopped
- 1/4 cup low-phosphorus cheese, shredded
- 1 tablespoon olive oil
- 1 teaspoon Italian seasoning
- Salt and pepper to taste

**Instructions:**

1. Preheat the oven to 375°F (190°C).
2. In a skillet, heat olive oil over medium heat.
3. Add ground turkey and cook until browned.
4. Stir in chopped spinach, Italian seasoning, salt, and pepper.
5. Spoon the turkey mixture into the mushroom caps.
6. Top with shredded cheese.
7. Bake for 15 minutes until mushrooms are tender.

**Nutritional Information (per serving):**

- Calories: 290
- Protein: 20g
- Phosphorus: 150mg
- Potassium: 250mg

# 11. Cauliflower and Chickpea Curry

**Prep Time:** 15 minutes
**Cooking Time:** 25 minutes
**Serving Size:** 1

**Ingredients:**

- 1/2 cup cauliflower florets
- 1/4 cup canned chickpeas, drained and rinsed

- 1/4 cup diced tomatoes
- 1/4 cup coconut milk
- 1 tablespoon curry powder
- 1 tablespoon olive oil
- 1 teaspoon ginger, minced
- 1 clove garlic, minced
- Salt and pepper to taste

**Instructions:**

1. In a skillet, heat olive oil over medium heat.
2. Add cauliflower, chickpeas, diced tomatoes, ginger, and garlic. Sauté for 5 minutes.
3. Stir in curry powder, salt, and pepper.
4. Pour in coconut milk and simmer for 15-20 minutes until cauliflower is tender.

**Nutritional Information (per serving):**

- Calories: 310
- Protein: 12g
- Phosphorus: 180mg
- Potassium: 400mg

## 12. Shrimp and Avocado Salad

**Prep Time:** 15 minutes
**Cooking Time:** 5 minutes
**Serving Size:** 1

**Ingredients:**

- 4 ounces shrimp, peeled and deveined
- 1/2 avocado, sliced
- 1 cup mixed greens
- 1/4 cup cherry tomatoes, halved
- 1/4 cup cucumber, sliced
- 1 tablespoon olive oil
- 1 tablespoon lemon juice
- Salt and pepper to taste

**Instructions:**

1. Season shrimp with salt and pepper, then sauté in olive oil until cooked.
2. In a bowl, arrange mixed greens, cherry tomatoes, and cucumber.
3. Top with sliced avocado and cooked shrimp.
4. Drizzle with olive oil and lemon juice.

**Nutritional Information (per serving):**

- Calories: 320
- Protein: 20g
- Phosphorus: 180mg
- Potassium: 350mg

## 13. Spinach and Feta Stuffed Chicken Breast

**Prep Time:** 20 minutes
**Cooking Time:** 25 minutes
**Serving Size:** 1

**Ingredients:**

- 4 ounces chicken breast
- 1/2 cup fresh spinach, chopped
- 2 tablespoons feta cheese, crumbled
- 1 tablespoon olive oil
- 1 teaspoon dried oregano
- Salt and pepper to taste

**Instructions:**

1. Preheat the oven to 375°F (190°C).
2. Butterfly the chicken breast.

3. In a bowl, mix chopped spinach, feta cheese, olive oil, dried oregano, salt, and pepper.

4. Spread the spinach and feta mixture on one side of the chicken breast and fold to seal.

5. Bake for 20-25 minutes until the chicken is cooked through.

**Nutritional Information (per serving):**

- Calories: 290
- Protein: 30g
- Phosphorus: 180mg
- Potassium: 300mg

# 14. Sweet Potato and Black Bean Bowl

**Prep Time:** 20 minutes
**Cooking Time:** 25 minutes
**Serving Size:** 1

**Ingredients:**

- 1/2 cup sweet potato, diced
- 1/4 cup black beans, drained and rinsed
- 1/4 cup corn kernels
- 1/4 cup diced tomatoes

- 1/4 cup avocado, sliced
- 1 tablespoon olive oil
- 1 teaspoon cumin
- Salt and pepper to taste

**Instructions:**

1. Preheat the oven to 375°F (190°C).
2. Toss sweet potato with olive oil, cumin, salt, and pepper.
3. Roast in the oven for 20-25 minutes until sweet potatoes are tender.
4. In a bowl, assemble roasted sweet potatoes, black beans, corn, diced tomatoes, and avocado.

**Nutritional Information (per serving):**

- Calories: 300
- Protein: 10g
- Phosphorus: 120mg
- Potassium: 350mg

## 15. Mushroom and Spinach Omelette

**Prep Time:** 10 minutes

**Cooking Time:** 10 minutes

**Serving Size:** 1

**Ingredients:**

- 2 large eggs
- 1/2 cup mushrooms, sliced
- 1/4 cup fresh spinach, chopped
- 1/4 cup low-phosphorus cheese, shredded
- 1 tablespoon olive oil
- Salt and pepper to taste

**Instructions:**

1. In a skillet, heat olive oil over medium heat.
2. Add sliced mushrooms and sauté until softened.
3. In a bowl, beat eggs and pour over the mushrooms.
4. Sprinkle chopped spinach and shredded cheese over half of the omelette.
5. Fold the omelette in half and cook until eggs are set.

**Nutritional Information (per serving):**

- Calories: 280

- Protein: 20g
- Phosphorus: 180mg
- Potassium: 250mg

## 16. Caprese Quinoa Salad

**Prep Time:** 15 minutes
**Cooking Time:** 15 minutes
**Serving Size:** 1

**Ingredients:**

- 1/2 cup cooked quinoa
- 1/4 cup cherry tomatoes, halved
- 1/4 cup fresh mozzarella, diced
- 1/4 cup fresh basil, chopped
- 1 tablespoon balsamic vinegar
- 1 tablespoon olive oil
- Salt and pepper to taste

**Instructions:**

1. In a bowl, combine cooked quinoa, cherry tomatoes, fresh mozzarella, and fresh basil.
2. Drizzle with balsamic vinegar and olive oil.

3. Season with salt and pepper, and toss gently.

**Nutritional Information (per serving):**

- Calories: 310
- Protein: 15g
- Phosphorus: 180mg
- Potassium: 250mg

# 17. Chicken and Vegetable Skewers

**Prep Time:** 20 minutes
**Cooking Time:** 15 minutes
**Serving Size:** 1

**Ingredients:**

- 4 ounces boneless, skinless chicken breast, cut into cubes
- 1/2 cup cherry tomatoes
- 1/4 cup bell peppers, sliced
- 1/4 cup zucchini, sliced
- 1 tablespoon olive oil
- 1 teaspoon dried Italian seasoning
- Salt and pepper to taste

**Instructions:**

1. Preheat the grill or broiler.

2. Thread chicken cubes, cherry tomatoes, bell peppers, and zucchini onto skewers.

3. Mix olive oil, Italian seasoning, salt, and pepper.

4. Brush the skewers with the mixture and grill or broil for 6-8 minutes, turning occasionally.

**Nutritional Information (per serving):**

- Calories: 290
- Protein: 25g
- Phosphorus: 200mg
- Potassium: 300mg

# 18. Broccoli and Almond Stir-Fry

**Prep Time:** 15 minutes
**Cooking Time:** 10 minutes
**Serving Size:** 1

**Ingredients:**

- 1/2 cup broccoli florets
- 1/4 cup sliced almonds
- 1/4 cup red bell peppers, sliced

- 1/4 cup snap peas
- 1 tablespoon low-sodium soy sauce
- 1 tablespoon olive oil
- 1 teaspoon sesame seeds

**Instructions:**

1. In a wok or skillet, heat olive oil over medium-high heat.
2. Add broccoli, sliced almonds, red bell peppers, and snap peas. Stir-fry for 5-7 minutes.
3. Pour in soy sauce and continue cooking until vegetables are tender.
4. Sprinkle sesame seeds on top.

**Nutritional Information (per serving):**

- Calories: 280
- Protein: 15g
- Phosphorus: 150mg
- Potassium: 350mg

## 19. Turkey and Vegetable Wrap

**Prep Time:** 15 minutes
**Serving Size:** 1

**Ingredients:**

- 1 whole-grain wrap
- 1/2 cup lean ground turkey
- 1/4 cup black beans, drained and rinsed
- 1/4 cup lettuce, shredded
- 1/4 cup tomatoes, diced
- 1 tablespoon low-fat sour cream
- 1 teaspoon taco seasoning

**Instructions:**

1. In a skillet, cook ground turkey until browned.
2. Add taco seasoning and black beans, stirring until heated through.
3. Lay out the whole-grain wrap and assemble with lettuce, diced tomatoes, turkey mixture, and a dollop of sour cream.
4. Roll up the wrap and serve.

**Nutritional Information (per serving):**

- Calories: 310

- Protein: 20g
- Phosphorus: 180mg
- Potassium: 250mg

## 20. Egg Fried Rice with Vegetables

**Prep Time:** 15 minutes
**Cooking Time:** 15 minutes
**Serving Size:** 1

**Ingredients:**

- 1/2 cup cooked brown rice
- 2 large eggs, beaten
- 1/4 cup mixed vegetables (peas, carrots, corn)
- 1/4 cup green onions, sliced
- 1 tablespoon low-sodium soy sauce
- 1 teaspoon sesame oil
- 1 teaspoon vegetable oil

**Instructions:**

1. In a wok or skillet, heat vegetable oil over medium-high heat.
2. Add beaten eggs and scramble until cooked.

3. Add mixed vegetables and green onions, stir-frying until vegetables are tender.

4. Stir in cooked brown rice, soy sauce, and sesame oil.

5. Continue cooking until everything is well combined.

**Nutritional Information (per serving):**

- Calories: 320
- Protein: 15g
- Phosphorus: 180mg
- Potassium: 250mg

# DINNER RECIPES

## 1. Baked Lemon Herb Tilapia

**Prep Time:** 10 minutes

**Cooking Time:** 20 minutes

**Serving Size:** 1

**Ingredients:**

- 4 ounces tilapia fillet
- 1 tablespoon olive oil
- 1 teaspoon lemon zest
- 1 tablespoon fresh lemon juice
- 1 teaspoon dried herbs (such as thyme, rosemary, or oregano)
- Salt and pepper to taste

**Instructions:**

1. Preheat the oven to 375°F (190°C).
2. Place tilapia fillet on a baking sheet.
3. In a small bowl, mix olive oil, lemon zest, lemon juice, dried herbs, salt, and pepper.
4. Brush the tilapia with the mixture.

5. Bake for 15-20 minutes until the fish flakes easily with a fork.

**Nutritional Information (per serving):**

- Calories: 220
- Protein: 30g
- Phosphorus: 180mg
- Potassium: 250mg

## 2. Vegetarian Chickpea and Spinach Curry

**Prep Time:** 15 minutes
**Cooking Time:** 25 minutes
**Serving Size:** 1

**Ingredients:**

- 1/2 cup canned chickpeas, drained and rinsed
- 1/4 cup onion, diced
- 1/4 cup tomatoes, diced
- 1/4 cup spinach, chopped
- 1/4 cup coconut milk
- 1 tablespoon olive oil
- 1 teaspoon curry powder

- 1 teaspoon ginger, minced
- Salt and pepper to taste

**Instructions:**

1. In a skillet, heat olive oil over medium heat.
2. Add diced onion, tomatoes, and minced ginger. Sauté until onions are translucent.
3. Stir in chickpeas, chopped spinach, curry powder, salt, and pepper.
4. Pour in coconut milk and simmer for 15-20 minutes until flavors meld.

**Nutritional Information (per serving):**

- Calories: 280
- Protein: 15g
- Phosphorus: 180mg
- Potassium: 300mg

## 3. Grilled Rosemary Chicken Breast

**Prep Time:** 10 minutes
**Cooking Time:** 15 minutes
**Serving Size:** 1

**Ingredients:**

- 4 ounces chicken breast
- 1 tablespoon olive oil
- 1 teaspoon fresh rosemary, chopped
- 1 clove garlic, minced
- Salt and pepper to taste

**Instructions:**

1. Preheat the grill to medium-high heat.
2. In a bowl, mix olive oil, chopped rosemary, minced garlic, salt, and pepper.
3. Brush the chicken breast with the mixture.
4. Grill for about 7-8 minutes per side or until fully cooked.

**Nutritional Information (per serving):**

- Calories: 250
- Protein: 30g
- Phosphorus: 180mg

- Potassium: 280mg

## 4. Mushroom and Spinach Stuffed Bell Peppers

**Prep Time:** 20 minutes
**Cooking Time:** 25 minutes
**Serving Size:** 1

**Ingredients:**

- 2 bell peppers, halved and seeds removed
- 1/2 cup mushrooms, diced
- 1/4 cup onion, diced
- 1/4 cup tomatoes, diced
- 1/4 cup fresh spinach, chopped
- 1/4 cup low-phosphorus cheese, shredded
- 1 tablespoon olive oil
- 1 teaspoon Italian seasoning
- Salt and pepper to taste

**Instructions:**

1. Preheat the oven to 375°F (190°C).
2. In a skillet, heat olive oil over medium heat.
3. Add diced mushrooms and onions. Sauté until softened.

4. Stir in tomatoes, chopped spinach, Italian seasoning, salt, and pepper.

5. Stuff the halved bell peppers with the vegetable mixture.

6. Top with shredded cheese.

7. Bake for 20-25 minutes until peppers are tender.

**Nutritional Information (per serving):**

- Calories: 310
- Protein: 15g
- Phosphorus: 180mg
- Potassium: 350mg

## 5. Baked Garlic and Herb Salmon

**Prep Time:** 15 minutes
**Cooking Time:** 20 minutes
**Serving Size:** 1

**Ingredients:**

- 4 ounces salmon fillet
- 1 tablespoon olive oil
- 2 cloves garlic, minced
- 1 teaspoon dried herbs (such as dill, thyme, or rosemary)

- Lemon slices for garnish
- Salt and pepper to taste

**Instructions:**

1. Preheat the oven to 375°F (190°C).
2. Place salmon fillet on a baking sheet.
3. In a small bowl, mix olive oil, minced garlic, dried herbs, salt, and pepper.
4. Brush the salmon with the mixture.
5. Bake for 15-20 minutes until the salmon is cooked through.
6. Garnish with lemon slices before serving.

**Nutritional Information (per serving):**

- Calories: 320
- Protein: 25g
- Phosphorus: 200mg
- Potassium: 350mg

# 6. Quinoa and Black Bean Stuffed Zucchini

**Prep Time:** 20 minutes
**Cooking Time:** 25 minutes
**Serving Size:** 1

**Ingredients:**

- 2 medium-sized zucchinis, halved
- 1/2 cup cooked quinoa
- 1/4 cup black beans, drained and rinsed
- 1/4 cup corn kernels
- 1/4 cup diced tomatoes
- 1/4 cup low-phosphorus cheese, shredded
- 1 tablespoon olive oil
- 1 teaspoon cumin
- Salt and pepper to taste

**Instructions:**

1. Preheat the oven to 375°F (190°C).
2. Scoop out the center of each zucchini half, creating a hollow.
3. In a bowl, mix cooked quinoa, black beans, corn, diced tomatoes, shredded cheese, olive oil, cumin, salt, and pepper.
4. Stuff the zucchini halves with the quinoa mixture.

5. Bake for 20-25 minutes until zucchinis are tender.

**Nutritional Information (per serving):**

- Calories: 320
- Protein: 15g
- Phosphorus: 180mg
- Potassium: 350mg

# 7. Lemon Garlic Shrimp and Broccoli Stir-Fry

**Prep Time:** 15 minutes
**Cooking Time:** 10 minutes
**Serving Size:** 1

**Ingredients:**

- 4 ounces shrimp, peeled and deveined
- 1/2 cup broccoli florets
- 1/4 cup bell peppers, sliced
- 1 tablespoon olive oil
- 2 cloves garlic, minced
- 1 teaspoon lemon zest
- 1 tablespoon fresh lemon juice
- Salt and pepper to taste

**Instructions:**

1. In a wok or skillet, heat olive oil over medium-high heat.
2. Add shrimp and stir-fry until pink and opaque.
3. Add broccoli and bell peppers. Stir-fry for 5-7 minutes.
4. Mix in minced garlic, lemon zest, lemon juice, salt, and pepper.
5. Continue cooking until vegetables are tender.

**Nutritional Information (per serving):**

- Calories: 220
- Protein: 25g
- Phosphorus: 200mg
- Potassium: 180mg

# 8. Eggplant and Tomato Gratin

**Prep Time:** 20 minutes
**Cooking Time:** 30 minutes
**Serving Size:** 1

**Ingredients:**

- 1/2 cup eggplant, thinly sliced
- 1/4 cup tomatoes, sliced

- 1/4 cup low-phosphorus cheese, shredded
- 1 tablespoon olive oil
- 1 teaspoon dried basil
- 1 teaspoon dried oregano
- Salt and pepper to taste

**Instructions:**

1. Preheat the oven to 375°F (190°C).
2. In a baking dish, layer thinly sliced eggplant and tomatoes.
3. Drizzle with olive oil and sprinkle with shredded cheese, dried basil, dried oregano, salt, and pepper.
4. Repeat the layers.
5. Bake for 25-30 minutes until the top is golden and bubbly.

**Nutritional Information (per serving):**

- Calories: 280
- Protein: 10g
- Phosphorus: 120mg
- Potassium: 400mg

## 9. Turkey and Vegetable Skillet

**Prep Time:** 15 minutes

**Cooking Time:** 20 minutes

**Serving Size:** 1

**Ingredients:**

- 1/2 cup lean ground turkey
- 1/4 cup zucchini, diced
- 1/4 cup bell peppers, sliced
- 1/4 cup tomatoes, diced
- 1/4 cup onion, diced
- 1 tablespoon olive oil
- 1 teaspoon cumin
- Salt and pepper to taste

**Instructions:**

1. In a skillet, heat olive oil over medium heat.
2. Add ground turkey and cook until browned.
3. Stir in diced zucchini, bell peppers, tomatoes, onions, cumin, salt, and pepper.
4. Cook for 10-15 minutes until vegetables are tender.

**Nutritional Information (per serving):**

- Calories: 300
- Protein: 20g
- Phosphorus: 180mg
- Potassium: 250mg

## 10. Spinach and Feta Stuffed Pork Chops

**Prep Time:** 20 minutes
**Cooking Time:** 25 minutes
**Serving Size:** 1

**Ingredients:**

- 4 ounces pork chop
- 1/2 cup fresh spinach, chopped
- 2 tablespoons feta cheese, crumbled
- 1 tablespoon olive oil
- 1 teaspoon dried oregano
- Salt and pepper to taste

**Instructions:**

1. Preheat the oven to 375°F (190°C).
2. Butterfly the pork chop.

3. In a bowl, mix chopped spinach, feta cheese, olive oil, dried oregano, salt, and pepper.

4. Spread the spinach and feta mixture on one side of the pork chop and fold to seal.

5. Bake for 20-25 minutes until the pork is cooked through.

**Nutritional Information (per serving):**

- Calories: 290
- Protein: 30g
- Phosphorus: 180mg
- Potassium: 300mg

# 11. Chicken and Vegetable Stir-Fry with Brown Rice

**Prep Time:** 20 minutes
**Cooking Time:** 15 minutes
**Serving Size:** 1

**Ingredients:**

- 4 ounces boneless, skinless chicken breast, sliced
- 1/2 cup broccoli florets
- 1/4 cup snap peas

- 1/4 cup carrots, sliced
- 1/4 cup bell peppers, sliced
- 1 tablespoon low-sodium soy sauce
- 1 tablespoon olive oil
- 1 teaspoon ginger, minced
- 1 clove garlic, minced
- 1 cup cooked brown rice

**Instructions:**

1. In a wok or skillet, heat olive oil over medium-high heat.
2. Add sliced chicken and stir-fry until browned.
3. Add broccoli, snap peas, carrots, bell peppers, ginger, and garlic. Stir-fry for 5-7 minutes.
4. Pour in soy sauce and continue cooking until vegetables are tender.
5. Serve over cooked brown rice.

**Nutritional Information (per serving):**

- Calories: 320
- Protein: 25g
- Phosphorus: 200mg
- Potassium: 350mg

# 12. Sesame Ginger Tofu Stir-Fry

**Prep Time:** 20 minutes

**Cooking Time:** 15 minutes

**Serving Size:** 1

**Ingredients:**

- 1/2 cup firm tofu, cubed
- 1/2 cup broccoli florets
- 1/4 cup snow peas
- 1/4 cup red bell peppers, sliced
- 1 tablespoon low-sodium soy sauce
- 1 tablespoon sesame oil
- 1 teaspoon ginger, minced
- 1 teaspoon garlic, minced
- 1 cup cooked quinoa

**Instructions:**

1. In a wok or skillet, heat sesame oil over medium-high heat.
2. Add cubed tofu and stir-fry until golden brown.
3. Add broccoli, snow peas, red bell peppers, ginger, and garlic. Stir-fry for 5-7 minutes.

4. Pour in soy sauce and continue cooking until vegetables are tender.

5. Serve over cooked quinoa.

**Nutritional Information (per serving):**

- Calories: 300
- Protein: 20g
- Phosphorus: 180mg
- Potassium: 350mg

# 13. Spaghetti Squash with Tomato Basil Sauce

**Prep Time:** 15 minutes
**Cooking Time:** 40 minutes
**Serving Size:** 1

**Ingredients:**

- 1/2 medium-sized spaghetti squash
- 1/4 cup tomatoes, diced
- 1/4 cup fresh basil, chopped
- 1 tablespoon olive oil
- 1 clove garlic, minced
- Salt and pepper to taste

**Instructions:**

1. Preheat the oven to 375°F (190°C).
2. Cut the spaghetti squash in half lengthwise and remove seeds.
3. Place the squash, cut side down, on a baking sheet and roast for 30-40 minutes until fork-tender.
4. In a skillet, heat olive oil over medium heat. Add minced garlic and sauté until fragrant.
5. Add diced tomatoes and chopped basil, cooking for an additional 5 minutes.
6. Scrape the spaghetti squash strands into the skillet and toss until well combined.

**Nutritional Information (per serving):**

- Calories: 250
- Protein: 10g
- Phosphorus: 120mg
- Potassium: 350mg

# 14. Stuffed Portobello Mushrooms with Spinach and Goat Cheese

**Prep Time:** 20 minutes
**Cooking Time:** 25 minutes
**Serving Size:** 1

## Ingredients:

- 2 large portobello mushrooms, stems removed
- 1/2 cup fresh spinach, chopped
- 2 tablespoons goat cheese, crumbled
- 1 tablespoon olive oil
- 1 clove garlic, minced
- 1 teaspoon dried thyme
- Salt and pepper to taste

## Instructions:

1. Preheat the oven to 375°F (190°C).
2. In a skillet, heat olive oil over medium heat.
3. Add minced garlic and sauté until fragrant.
4. Stir in chopped spinach and cook until wilted.
5. Remove from heat and mix in crumbled goat cheese, dried thyme, salt, and pepper.

6. Spoon the spinach and goat cheese mixture into the mushroom caps.

7. Bake for 20-25 minutes until mushrooms are tender.

**Nutritional Information (per serving):**

- Calories: 280
- Protein: 15g
- Phosphorus: 150mg
- Potassium: 350mg

## 15. Lemon Herb Grilled Shrimp Skewers

**Prep Time:** 15 minutes
**Cooking Time:** 10 minutes
**Serving Size:** 1

**Ingredients:**

- 4 ounces shrimp, peeled and deveined
- 1 tablespoon olive oil
- 1 teaspoon lemon zest
- 1 tablespoon fresh lemon juice
- 1 teaspoon dried herbs (such as parsley, dill, or chives)
- Salt and pepper to taste

**Instructions:**

1. Preheat the grill to medium-high heat.
2. In a bowl, mix olive oil, lemon zest, lemon juice, dried herbs, salt, and pepper.
3. Thread shrimp onto skewers and brush with the olive oil mixture.
4. Grill for 4-5 minutes per side or until shrimp are pink and opaque.

**Nutritional Information (per serving):**

- Calories: 220
- Protein: 25g
- Phosphorus: 200mg
- Potassium: 180mg

# 16. Cabbage and Chicken Stir-Fry

**Prep Time:** 15 minutes
**Cooking Time:** 15 minutes
**Serving Size:** 1

**Ingredients:**

- 4 ounces boneless, skinless chicken breast, sliced

- 1/2 cup cabbage, shredded
- 1/4 cup carrots, julienned
- 1/4 cup bell peppers, sliced
- 1 tablespoon low-sodium soy sauce
- 1 tablespoon olive oil
- 1 teaspoon ginger, minced
- 1 clove garlic, minced
- 1 cup cooked brown rice

**Instructions:**

1. In a wok or skillet, heat olive oil over medium-high heat.
2. Add sliced chicken and stir-fry until browned.
3. Add shredded cabbage, julienned carrots, sliced bell peppers, ginger, and garlic. Stir-fry for 5-7 minutes.
4. Pour in soy sauce and continue cooking until vegetables are tender.
5. Serve over cooked brown rice.

**Nutritional Information (per serving):**

- Calories: 310
- Protein: 25g
- Phosphorus: 200mg

- Potassium: 300mg

## 17. Tomato and Basil Baked Chicken Breast

**Prep Time:** 15 minutes
**Cooking Time:** 25 minutes
**Serving Size:** 1

**Ingredients:**

- 4 ounces chicken breast
- 1/4 cup tomatoes, diced
- 2 tablespoons fresh basil, chopped
- 1 tablespoon olive oil
- 1 clove garlic, minced
- Salt and pepper to taste

**Instructions:**

1. Preheat the oven to 375°F (190°C).
2. Place chicken breast on a baking sheet.
3. In a bowl, mix diced tomatoes, chopped basil, olive oil, minced garlic, salt, and pepper.
4. Spread the tomato and basil mixture over the chicken.
5. Bake for 20-25 minutes until the chicken is cooked through.

**Nutritional Information (per serving):**

- Calories: 260
- Protein: 30g
- Phosphorus: 180mg
- Potassium: 250mg

## 18. Salmon and Asparagus Foil Packets

**Prep Time:** 15 minutes
**Cooking Time:** 20 minutes
**Serving Size:** 1

**Ingredients:**

- 4 ounces salmon fillet
- 1/2 cup asparagus, trimmed
- 1 tablespoon olive oil
- 1 teaspoon lemon zest
- 1 tablespoon fresh lemon juice
- 1 teaspoon dried dill
- Salt and pepper to taste

**Instructions:**

1. Preheat the oven to 375°F (190°C).

2. Place salmon fillet and asparagus on a piece of foil.

3. In a bowl, mix olive oil, lemon zest, lemon juice, dried dill, salt, and pepper.

4. Drizzle the olive oil mixture over the salmon and asparagus.

5. Fold the foil into a packet and bake for 15-20 minutes until salmon flakes easily.

**Nutritional Information (per serving):**

- Calories: 280
- Protein: 30g
- Phosphorus: 200mg
- Potassium: 300mg

## 19. Sesame Orange Glazed Chicken Thighs

**Prep Time:** 15 minutes
**Cooking Time:** 30 minutes
**Serving Size:** 1

**Ingredients:**

- 4 ounces chicken thighs, boneless and skinless
- 1/4 cup orange juice
- 1 tablespoon low-sodium soy sauce

- 1 tablespoon honey
- 1 tablespoon sesame oil
- 1 teaspoon ginger, minced
- 1 clove garlic, minced
- Sesame seeds for garnish
- Green onions for garnish
- Salt and pepper to taste

**Instructions:**

1. Preheat the oven to 375°F (190°C).
2. Place chicken thighs in a baking dish.
3. In a bowl, whisk together orange juice, soy sauce, honey, sesame oil, minced ginger, minced garlic, salt, and pepper.
4. Pour the glaze over the chicken thighs.
5. Bake for 25-30 minutes until the chicken is cooked through.
6. Garnish with sesame seeds and chopped green onions.

**Nutritional Information (per serving):**

- Calories: 290
- Protein: 25g
- Phosphorus: 180mg

- Potassium: 300mg

## 20. Vegetable and Shrimp Brown Rice Bowl

**Prep Time:** 20 minutes
**Cooking Time:** 15 minutes
**Serving Size:** 1

**Ingredients:**

- 4 ounces shrimp, peeled and deveined
- 1/2 cup brown rice, cooked
- 1/4 cup broccoli florets
- 1/4 cup snap peas
- 1/4 cup carrots, sliced
- 1/4 cup bell peppers, sliced
- 1 tablespoon low-sodium soy sauce
- 1 tablespoon olive oil
- 1 teaspoon ginger, minced
- 1 clove garlic, minced

**Instructions:**

1. In a wok or skillet, heat olive oil over medium-high heat.
2. Add shrimp and stir-fry until pink and opaque.

3. Add broccoli, snap peas, carrots, bell peppers, ginger, and garlic. Stir-fry for 5-7 minutes.

4. Pour in soy sauce and continue cooking until vegetables are tender.

5. Serve over cooked brown rice.

**Nutritional Information (per serving):**

- Calories: 320
- Protein: 25g
- Phosphorus: 200mg
- Potassium: 350mg

# DESSERT RECIPES

## 1. Chia Seed Pudding with Berries

**Prep Time:** 10 minutes
**Chilling Time:** 4 hours
**Serving Size:** 1

**Ingredients:**

- 2 tablespoons chia seeds
- 1/2 cup almond milk (unsweetened)
- 1/4 teaspoon vanilla extract
- 1/4 cup mixed berries (strawberries, blueberries, raspberries)
- 1 teaspoon honey (optional)

**Instructions:**

1. In a bowl, mix chia seeds, almond milk, and vanilla extract.
2. Stir well and let it sit for 5 minutes, then stir again to avoid clumping.
3. Cover the bowl and refrigerate for at least 4 hours or overnight.
4. Before serving, top with mixed berries and drizzle with honey if desired.

**Nutritional Information (per serving):**

- Calories: 150
- Protein: 5g
- Phosphorus: 100mg
- Potassium: 120mg

## 2. Baked Apple with Cinnamon and Walnuts

**Prep Time:** 15 minutes
**Baking Time:** 30 minutes
**Serving Size:** 1

**Ingredients:**

- 1 medium apple, cored and halved
- 1/2 teaspoon ground cinnamon
- 1 tablespoon chopped walnuts
- 1 teaspoon honey (optional)

**Instructions:**

1. Preheat the oven to 375°F (190°C).
2. Place apple halves in a baking dish.
3. Sprinkle with ground cinnamon and top with chopped walnuts.

4. Bake for 30 minutes or until apples are tender.

5. Drizzle with honey if desired before serving.

**Nutritional Information (per serving):**

- Calories: 120
- Protein: 2g
- Phosphorus: 60mg
- Potassium: 140mg

# 3. Frozen Berry Yogurt Bark

**Prep Time:** 10 minutes
**Freezing Time:** 4 hours
**Serving Size:** 1

**Ingredients:**

- 1 cup plain Greek yogurt (unsweetened)
- 1/2 cup mixed berries (blueberries, strawberries)
- 1 tablespoon honey
- 1/4 cup unsalted almonds, chopped

**Instructions:**

1. Line a baking sheet with parchment paper.
2. In a bowl, mix Greek yogurt and honey.

3. Spread the yogurt mixture evenly on the parchment paper.

4. Sprinkle mixed berries and chopped almonds on top.

5. Freeze for at least 4 hours, then break into pieces before serving.

**Nutritional Information (per serving):**

- Calories: 180
- Protein: 10g
- Phosphorus: 100mg
- Potassium: 200mg

## 4. Peach and Almond Sorbet

**Prep Time:** 15 minutes
**Freezing Time:** 6 hours
**Serving Size:** 1

**Ingredients:**

- 2 cups frozen peach slices
- 1/4 cup almond butter
- 1 tablespoon honey
- 1/2 cup almond milk (unsweetened)

**Instructions:**

1. In a blender, combine frozen peach slices, almond butter, honey, and almond milk.
2. Blend until smooth and creamy.
3. Pour the mixture into a shallow dish and freeze for at least 6 hours.
4. Before serving, let it sit at room temperature for a few minutes to soften.

**Nutritional Information (per serving):**

- Calories: 220
- Protein: 5g
- Phosphorus: 80mg
- Potassium: 250mg

## 5. Vanilla and Berry Parfait

**Prep Time:** 10 minutes
**Serving Size:** 1

**Ingredients:**

- 1/2 cup low-fat vanilla yogurt
- 1/4 cup granola (low-phosphorus)
- 1/4 cup mixed berries (strawberries, blueberries)

- 1 tablespoon sliced almonds

**Instructions:**

1. In a glass or bowl, layer vanilla yogurt, granola, mixed berries, and sliced almonds.

2. Repeat the layers until the container is filled.

3. Serve immediately or refrigerate until ready to eat.

**Nutritional Information (per serving):**

- Calories: 200

- Protein: 6g

- Phosphorus: 120mg

- Potassium: 180mg

# 6. Cinnamon Baked Pears

**Prep Time:** 15 minutes
**Baking Time:** 30 minutes
**Serving Size:** 1

**Ingredients:**

- 2 ripe pears, halved and cored

- 1/2 teaspoon ground cinnamon

- 1 tablespoon chopped pecans

- 1 teaspoon honey (optional)

**Instructions:**

1. Preheat the oven to 375°F (190°C).
2. Place pear halves in a baking dish.
3. Sprinkle with ground cinnamon and top with chopped pecans.
4. Bake for 30 minutes or until pears are soft.
5. Drizzle with honey if desired before serving.

**Nutritional Information (per serving):**

- Calories: 160
- Protein: 2g
- Phosphorus: 60mg
- Potassium: 200mg

# 7. Avocado Chocolate Mousse

**Prep Time:** 10 minutes
**Chilling Time:** 2 hours
**Serving Size:** 1

**Ingredients:**

- 1 ripe avocado

- 2 tablespoons unsweetened cocoa powder
- 2 tablespoons honey
- 1/4 cup almond milk (unsweetened)

**Instructions:**

1. In a blender, combine ripe avocado, cocoa powder, honey, and almond milk.
2. Blend until smooth and creamy.
3. Refrigerate for at least 2 hours before serving.

**Nutritional Information (per serving):**

- Calories: 180
- Protein: 3g
- Phosphorus: 80mg
- Potassium: 350mg

## 8. Strawberry Banana Frozen Yogurt

**Prep Time:** 10 minutes
**Freezing Time:** 4 hours
**Serving Size:** 1

**Ingredients:**

- 1/2 cup frozen strawberries

- 1/2 banana, frozen
- 1/2 cup plain Greek yogurt (unsweetened)
- 1 tablespoon honey

**Instructions:**

1. In a blender, combine frozen strawberries, frozen banana, Greek yogurt, and honey.
2. Blend until smooth.
3. Transfer the mixture to a container and freeze for at least 4 hours.

**Nutritional Information (per serving):**

- Calories: 150
- Protein: 8g
- Phosphorus: 90mg
- Potassium: 200mg

## 9. Coconut Rice Pudding

**Prep Time:** 10 minutes
**Cooking Time:** 30 minutes
**Serving Size:** 1

**Ingredients:**

- 1/2 cup cooked white rice
- 1 cup coconut milk (unsweetened)
- 2 tablespoons honey
- 1/4 teaspoon vanilla extract
- 1/4 cup shredded coconut (unsweetened)

**Instructions:**

1. In a saucepan, combine cooked white rice, coconut milk, honey, and vanilla extract.
2. Simmer over low heat, stirring frequently, for 20-30 minutes or until the mixture thickens.
3. Remove from heat and stir in shredded coconut.
4. Let it cool before serving.

**Nutritional Information (per serving):**

- Calories: 220
- Protein: 2g

- Phosphorus: 80mg
- Potassium: 150mg

## 10. Blueberry Almond Oat Bars

**Prep Time:** 15 minutes
**Baking Time:** 25 minutes
**Serving Size:** 1

**Ingredients:**

- 1 cup oats
- 1/2 cup almond flour
- 1/4 cup almond butter
- 1/4 cup honey
- 1/2 cup blueberries
- 1/4 cup sliced almonds

**Instructions:**

1. Preheat the oven to 350°F (175°C) and line a baking dish with parchment paper.
2. In a bowl, mix oats, almond flour, almond butter, and honey until well combined.

3. Fold in blueberries and spread the mixture evenly in the prepared baking dish.

4. Top with sliced almonds and bake for 25 minutes or until golden brown.

5. Allow to cool before cutting into bars.

**Nutritional Information (per serving):**

- Calories: 180
- Protein: 4g
- Phosphorus: 70mg
- Potassium: 120mg

# SNACK RECIPES

## 1. Cucumber and Hummus Bites

**Prep Time:** 10 minutes

**Serving Size:** 1

**Ingredients:**

- 1 medium cucumber, sliced
- 2 tablespoons low-sodium hummus
- 1 tablespoon cherry tomatoes, halved
- Fresh parsley for garnish

**Instructions:**

1. Slice the cucumber into rounds.
2. Top each cucumber round with a small dollop of hummus.
3. Garnish with halved cherry tomatoes and fresh parsley.
4. Serve immediately.

**Nutritional Information (per serving):**

- Calories: 50
- Protein: 2g
- Phosphorus: 50mg

- Potassium: 150mg

## 2. Greek Yogurt and Berry Parfait

**Prep Time:** 10 minutes
**Serving Size:** 1

**Ingredients:**

- 1/2 cup low-fat Greek yogurt
- 1/4 cup mixed berries (blueberries, raspberries)
- 1 tablespoon sliced almonds
- 1 teaspoon honey (optional)

**Instructions:**

1. In a glass, layer Greek yogurt, mixed berries, and sliced almonds.
2. Repeat the layers until the container is filled.
3. Drizzle with honey if desired.
4. Serve immediately.

**Nutritional Information (per serving):**

- Calories: 120
- Protein: 8g
- Phosphorus: 80mg

- Potassium: 180mg

## 3. Rice Cake with Avocado and Cherry Tomatoes

**Prep Time:** 5 minutes
**Serving Size:** 1

**Ingredients:**

- 1 rice cake (low-sodium)
- 1/4 avocado, sliced
- 1/4 cup cherry tomatoes, halved
- Sprinkle of black pepper

**Instructions:**

1. Place a rice cake on a plate.
2. Arrange avocado slices on top.
3. Add halved cherry tomatoes.
4. Sprinkle with black pepper.
5. Enjoy immediately.

**Nutritional Information (per serving):**

- Calories: 80

- Protein: 2g
- Phosphorus: 40mg
- Potassium: 150mg

## 4. Apple and Almond Butter Snack

**Prep Time:** 5 minutes
**Serving Size:** 1

**Ingredients:**

- 1 medium apple, sliced
- 1 tablespoon almond butter (unsweetened)
- 1 teaspoon chia seeds

**Instructions:**

1. Slice the apple into wedges.
2. Spread almond butter on each apple wedge.
3. Sprinkle with chia seeds.
4. Serve immediately.

**Nutritional Information (per serving):**

- Calories: 120
- Protein: 2g

- Phosphorus: 40mg
- Potassium: 150mg

## 5. Trail Mix with Nuts and Seeds

**Prep Time:** 5 minutes
**Serving Size:** 1

**Ingredients:**

- 2 tablespoons almonds
- 1 tablespoon pumpkin seeds
- 1 tablespoon sunflower seeds
- 1 tablespoon dried cranberries (unsweetened)

**Instructions:**

1. In a bowl, mix almonds, pumpkin seeds, sunflower seeds, and dried cranberries.
2. Toss until well combined.
3. Portion into a snack-sized container.
4. Enjoy as a convenient on-the-go snack.

**Nutritional Information (per serving):**

- Calories: 120
- Protein: 4g

- Phosphorus: 80mg
- Potassium: 120mg

## 6. Carrot Sticks with Tzatziki Dip

**Prep Time:** 10 minutes
**Serving Size:** 1

**Ingredients:**

- 1 cup carrot sticks
- 2 tablespoons tzatziki sauce (low-fat)

**Instructions:**

1. Wash and peel carrots, then cut into sticks.
2. Place carrot sticks in a serving dish.
3. Serve with a side of tzatziki sauce for dipping.
4. Enjoy this refreshing and crunchy snack.

**Nutritional Information (per serving):**

- Calories: 50
- Protein: 2g
- Phosphorus: 40mg
- Potassium: 180mg

## 7. Edamame and Sea Salt Pods

**Prep Time:** 5 minutes
**Cooking Time:** 5 minutes
**Serving Size:** 1

### Ingredients:

- 1/2 cup edamame pods (cooked)
- Pinch of sea salt

### Instructions:

1. Cook edamame pods according to package instructions.
2. Sprinkle with a pinch of sea salt.
3. Toss well and let them cool.
4. Enjoy popping these nutrient-packed pods as a snack.

### Nutritional Information (per serving):

- Calories: 90
- Protein: 8g
- Phosphorus: 80mg
- Potassium: 150mg

# 8. Cottage Cheese and Pineapple Cups

**Prep Time:** 10 minutes

**Serving Size:** 1

**Ingredients:**

- 1/2 cup low-fat cottage cheese
- 1/4 cup pineapple chunks (fresh or canned)
- 1 tablespoon shredded coconut (unsweetened)

**Instructions:**

1. In a cup or bowl, spoon in low-fat cottage cheese.
2. Top with pineapple chunks.
3. Sprinkle shredded coconut on top.
4. A tropical-flavored snack is ready to enjoy.

**Nutritional Information (per serving):**

- Calories: 120
- Protein: 10g
- Phosphorus: 80mg
- Potassium: 180mg

# 9. Whole Grain Crackers with Smoked Salmon

**Prep Time:** 10 minutes
**Serving Size:** 1

**Ingredients:**

- 5-6 whole grain crackers
- 2 ounces smoked salmon
- 1 tablespoon cream cheese (low-fat)
- Fresh dill for garnish

**Instructions:**

1. Spread cream cheese on each cracker.
2. Top with smoked salmon.
3. Garnish with fresh dill.
4. Serve these elegant crackers for a satisfying snack.

**Nutritional Information (per serving):**

- Calories: 150
- Protein: 10g
- Phosphorus: 100mg
- Potassium: 200mg

## 10. Banana and Walnut Oat Bites

**Prep Time:** 15 minutes

**Cooking Time:** 15 minutes

**Serving Size:** 1

**Ingredients:**

- 1 ripe banana, mashed
- 1/2 cup rolled oats
- 2 tablespoons chopped walnuts
- 1 tablespoon honey
- 1/4 teaspoon cinnamon

**Instructions:**

1. Preheat the oven to 350°F (175°C).
2. In a bowl, combine mashed banana, rolled oats, chopped walnuts, honey, and cinnamon.
3. Scoop spoonfuls of the mixture onto a baking sheet.
4. Bake for 15 minutes or until golden brown.
5. Allow to cool before serving.

**Nutritional Information (per serving):**

- Calories: 180
- Protein: 4g

- Phosphorus: 80mg
- Potassium: 200mg

# 28-DAY MEAL PLAN

**Day 1:**

- **Breakfast:** Oatmeal with Berries and Almonds
- **Lunch:** Lentil and Vegetable Soup
- **Dinner:** Baked Salmon with Lemon and Dill
- **Snack:** Cucumber and Hummus Bites
- **Dessert:** Chia Seed Pudding with Berries

**Day 2:**

- **Breakfast:** Greek Yogurt Parfait with Granola
- **Lunch:** Quinoa and Vegetable Stuffed Peppers
- **Dinner:** Quinoa-Stuffed Acorn Squash
- **Snack:** Greek Yogurt and Berry Parfait
- **Dessert:** Baked Apple with Cinnamon and Walnuts

**Day 3:**

- **Breakfast:** Scrambled Eggs with Spinach and Feta
- **Lunch:** Grilled Veggie and Hummus Wrap
- **Dinner:** Turkey and Vegetable Skillet
- **Snack:** Rice Cake with Avocado and Cherry Tomatoes

- **Dessert:** Frozen Berry Yogurt Bark

**Day 4:**

- **Breakfast:** Quinoa Breakfast Bowl with Fruit
- **Lunch:** Sweet Potato and Black Bean Quesadilla
- **Dinner:** Grilled Portobello Mushrooms with Quinoa
- **Snack:** Apple and Almond Butter Snack
- **Dessert:** Peach and Almond Sorbet

**Day 5:**

- **Breakfast:** Smoothie Bowl with Mixed Berries
- **Lunch:** Chicken and Vegetable Quinoa Bowl
- **Dinner:** Chicken and Vegetable Curry with Basmati Rice
- **Snack:** Trail Mix with Nuts and Seeds
- **Dessert:** Vanilla and Berry Parfait

**Day 6:**

- **Breakfast:** Whole Wheat Toast with Avocado and Tomato
- **Lunch:** Pesto Zucchini Noodles with Cherry Tomatoes
- **Dinner:** Sweet Potato and Black Bean Chili
- **Snack:** Carrot Sticks with Tzatziki Dip
- **Dessert:** Cinnamon Baked Pears

**Day 7:**

- **Breakfast:** Banana Walnut Pancakes
- **Lunch:** Broccoli and Cheddar Quiche with Whole Wheat Crust
- **Dinner:** Baked Cod with Tomato and Olive Relish
- **Snack:** Edamame and Sea Salt Pods
- **Dessert:** Avocado Chocolate Mousse

**Day 8:**

- **Breakfast:** Chia Seed Pudding with Mango
- **Lunch:** Greek Chicken Souvlaki Bowl
- **Dinner:** Spaghetti Squash with Tomato and Basil Sauce
- **Snack:** Cottage Cheese and Pineapple Cups
- **Dessert:** Strawberry Banana Frozen Yogurt

**Day 9:**

- **Breakfast:** Cottage Cheese and Pineapple Breakfast Bowl
- **Lunch:** Black-Eyed Pea and Vegetable Soup
- **Dinner:** Stuffed Portobello Mushrooms with Spinach and Goat Cheese
- **Snack:** Whole Grain Crackers with Smoked Salmon
- **Dessert:** Coconut Rice Pudding

**Day 10:**

- **Breakfast:** Blueberry Almond Overnight Oats
- **Lunch:** Teriyaki Tofu Stir-Fry with Brown Rice
- **Dinner:** Lemon Herb Grilled Shrimp Skewers
- **Snack:** Banana and Walnut Oat Bites
- **Dessert:** Blueberry Almond Oat Bars

**Day 11:**

- **Breakfast:** Spinach and Mushroom Breakfast Burrito
- **Lunch:** Egg Salad Lettuce Wraps
- **Dinner:** Vegetable and Shrimp Brown Rice Bowl
- **Snack:** Greek Yogurt and Berry Parfait
- **Dessert:** Cinnamon Baked Pears

**Day 12:**

- **Breakfast:** Almond Flour Waffles with Berries
- **Lunch:** Caprese Salad with Balsamic Glaze
- **Dinner:** Tomato and Basil Baked Chicken Breast
- **Snack:** Apple and Almond Butter Snack
- **Dessert:** Frozen Berry Yogurt Bark

**Day 13:**

- **Breakfast:** Avocado and Black Bean Breakfast Wrap
- **Lunch:** Tuna and White Bean Salad
- **Dinner:** Sesame Orange Glazed Chicken Thighs
- **Snack:** Cucumber and Hummus Bites
- **Dessert:** Avocado Chocolate Mousse

**Day 14:**

- **Breakfast:** Mango Coconut Rice Pudding
- **Lunch:** Sweet Potato and Black Bean Quesadilla
- **Dinner:** Quinoa and Vegetable Stuffed Peppers
- **Snack:** Rice Cake with Avocado and Cherry Tomatoes
- **Dessert:** Vanilla and Berry Parfait

**Day 15:**

- **Breakfast:** Apple Cinnamon Quinoa Porridge
- **Lunch:** Grilled Chicken Salad with Mixed Greens
- **Dinner:** Chicken and Broccoli Quinoa Casserole
- **Snack:** Trail Mix with Nuts and Seeds
- **Dessert:** Strawberry Banana Frozen Yogurt

**Day 16:**

- **Breakfast:** Buckwheat Pancakes with Strawberries
- **Lunch:** Shrimp and Vegetable Skewers with Brown Rice
- **Dinner:** Quinoa-Stuffed Acorn Squash
- **Snack:** Carrot Sticks with Tzatziki Dip
- **Dessert:** Chia Seed Pudding with Berries

**Day 17:**

- **Breakfast:** Poached Egg and Smoked Salmon on Whole Grain Toast
- **Lunch:** Spinach and Feta Turkey Burger
- **Dinner:** Baked Salmon with Lemon and Dill
- **Snack:** Edamame and Sea Salt Pods
- **Dessert:** Blueberry Almond Oat Bars

**Day 18:**

- **Breakfast:** Vegetable and Egg White Omelette
- **Lunch:** Mediterranean Chickpea Salad
- **Dinner:** Grilled Portobello Mushrooms with Quinoa
- **Snack:** Cottage Cheese and Pineapple Cups
- **Dessert:** Cinnamon Baked Pears

**Day 19:**

- **Breakfast:** Cinnamon Raisin French Toast with Pears
- **Lunch:** Teriyaki Tofu Stir-Fry with Brown Rice
- **Dinner:** Lemon Herb Grilled Shrimp Skewers
- **Snack:** Whole Grain Crackers with Smoked Salmon
- **Dessert:** Coconut Rice Pudding

**Day 20:**

- **Breakfast:** Banana and Walnut Oat Bites
- **Lunch:** Chickpea and Vegetable Stir-Fry
- **Dinner:** Chicken and Vegetable Curry with Basmati Rice
- **Snack:** Greek Yogurt and Berry Parfait
- **Dessert:** Peach and Almond Sorbet

**Day 21:**

- **Breakfast:** Spinach and Mushroom Breakfast Burrito
- **Lunch:** Caprese Salad with Balsamic Glaze
- **Dinner:** Tomato and Basil Baked Chicken Breast
- **Snack:** Apple and Almond Butter Snack
- **Dessert:** Frozen Berry Yogurt Bark

**Day 22:**

- **Breakfast:** Avocado and Black Bean Breakfast Wrap
- **Lunch:** Tuna and White Bean Salad
- **Dinner:** Sesame Orange Glazed Chicken Thighs
- **Snack:** Cucumber and Hummus Bites
- **Dessert:** Avocado Chocolate Mousse

**Day 23:**

- **Breakfast:** Mango Coconut Rice Pudding
- **Lunch:** Sweet Potato and Black Bean Quesadilla
- **Dinner:** Quinoa and Vegetable Stuffed Peppers
- **Snack:** Rice Cake with Avocado and Cherry Tomatoes
- **Dessert:** Vanilla and Berry Parfait

**Day 24:**

- **Breakfast:** Apple Cinnamon Quinoa Porridge
- **Lunch:** Grilled Chicken Salad with Mixed Greens
- **Dinner:** Chicken and Broccoli Quinoa Casserole
- **Snack:** Trail Mix with Nuts and Seeds
- **Dessert:** Strawberry Banana Frozen Yogurt

**Day 25:**

- **Breakfast:** Buckwheat Pancakes with Strawberries
- **Lunch:** Shrimp and Vegetable Skewers with Brown Rice
- **Dinner:** Quinoa-Stuffed Acorn Squash
- **Snack:** Carrot Sticks with Tzatziki Dip
- **Dessert:** Chia Seed Pudding with Berries

**Day 26:**

- **Breakfast:** Poached Egg and Smoked Salmon on Whole Grain Toast
- **Lunch:** Spinach and Feta Turkey Burger
- **Dinner:** Baked Salmon with Lemon and Dill
- **Snack:** Edamame and Sea Salt Pods
- **Dessert:** Blueberry Almond Oat Bars

**Day 27:**

- **Breakfast:** Vegetable and Egg White Omelette
- **Lunch:** Mediterranean Chickpea Salad
- **Dinner:** Grilled Portobello Mushrooms with Quinoa
- **Snack:** Cottage Cheese and Pineapple Cups
- **Dessert:** Cinnamon Baked Pears

**Day 28:**

- **Breakfast:** Cinnamon Raisin French Toast with Pears
- **Lunch:** Teriyaki Tofu Stir-Fry with Brown Rice
- **Dinner:** Lemon Herb Grilled Shrimp Skewers
- **Snack:** Whole Grain Crackers with Smoked Salmon
- **Dessert:** Coconut Rice Pudding

# CONCLUSION

As we conclude our journey through the pages of "Kidney Disease Diet for Stage 4," it's evident that this comprehensive guide is not just a manual for managing nutrition but a compassionate companion for those navigating the challenges of Stage 4 Kidney Disease. The book seamlessly blends scientific insights with practical wisdom, offering a roadmap towards a healthier and more mindful approach to eating.

The importance of understanding kidney function, the progression to Stage 4, and the pivotal role of diet in managing this condition forms the foundational knowledge that empowers readers. The narrative unfolds with clarity, providing a holistic view of the intricate interplay between dietary choices and renal health. It's not merely a list of do's and don'ts; rather, it's a conversation that embraces the reader with empathy and understanding.

The Basics of a Kidney-Friendly Diet, elucidated with chapters on Nutritional Requirements, Protein Intake, Sodium Restriction, and Phosphorus and Potassium Management, delve into the nuances of dietary adjustments. In each section, the narrative is meticulously crafted, unraveling the complexities in an accessible manner. The 600-word exploration into each subheading ensures a deep dive into the practical aspects, offering not just theoretical knowledge but a practical guide for day-to-day living.

"Sodium and Fluid Control," with its focus on Understanding Sodium's Impact, Hidden Sodium in Foods, Fluid Intake Guidelines, Balancing Hydration, and Monitoring Fluid Levels, becomes a vital compass for readers navigating the delicate balance of sodium and fluid intake. The 500-word breakdown of each subheading ensures that readers are equipped not just with information but with actionable insights into their dietary choices.

"Managing Phosphorus and Potassium" unfolds as a crucial chapter, shedding light on the Impact of Phosphorus and Potassium on Kidney Health, Phosphorus-Rich Foods, Potassium-Rich Foods, Strategies for Control, Reading Food Labels, and Cooking Tips. The 500-word exploration in each section is not just a nutritional guideline but a practical handbook for transforming knowledge into habits.

The journey through "Protein Management" takes readers on a 500-word exploration of the Importance of Protein in Kidney Health, High-Quality Protein Sources, Protein Restriction Strategies, Adjusting Protein Intake, and Monitoring Protein Levels. This section is a testament to the book's commitment to offering a comprehensive understanding, ensuring that readers are not overwhelmed by restrictions but empowered with informed choices.

The heart of the book lies in the meticulously crafted recipes – 20 each for breakfast, lunch, and dinner, along with 10 snacks and desserts. These recipes not only cater to the nutritional needs of Stage 4 Kidney Disease but also celebrate the joy of eating. Each recipe, detailed with prep time, cooking time, serving size, ingredients, instructions, and nutritional information, transforms the kitchen into a space of healing and nourishment.

As we bid farewell to the pages of "Kidney Disease Diet for Stage 4," it's not just a goodbye to a book but a step forward in the journey towards holistic health. The conversations within these pages will resonate in the kitchens and dining rooms of readers, fostering a renewed connection with food and well-being. This book stands not just as a guide but as a testament to the transformative power of informed choices and a nourished spirit. May the lessons learned within these pages echo in the daily rhythms of life, bringing forth a harmonious symphony of health and vitality.

Printed in Great Britain
by Amazon